LIVING ON H

CHANGE YOUR BODY – CHANGE YOU
TO
CHANGE YOUR LIFE & LIVE ON HIGH SPEED

MW01504059

A Raw and Vegan Wellness Guide
Includes High Speed Recipes and The Vortex Zone Wellness Plan

By

Scott Black

www.livingonhighspeed.com

Living On High Speed Online

Visit the Living On High Speed webpage at www.livingonhighspeed.com to become part of the online wellness community and receive support, updates and additional wellness resources.

Tell Us Your Story

We are interested in your experiences using the Living On High Speed Wellness Guide's programs and information as part of your personal journey. Your story of beginning or improving your healthy lifestyle may provide hope and inspiration for others. Please email your detailed personal experiences to getfit@coachscottblack.com.
Please provide your full name and contact information (email and /or phone number). Thank you.

Edited by Barbara Ault Black
Cover art by Scott A. Black, Barbara Ault Black and Tom Korba

Disclaimer: The following information is intended for general information purposes only. Individuals should consult with their health care provider before starting any diet plan or utilizing any information or programs presented in this book. Personal application of the material(s) set forth in this book is at the reader's discretion and is his or her sole responsibility.

ISBN-13: 978-1463618339
ISBN-10: 1463618336

Dedication

To my mother Loretta and to the millions of others who have lost the battle with cancer. I will continue to work in your honor to ensure future generations have a healthier outcome.

To the thousands of loyal Vita-Mix customers who watched my wellness seminars and asked for more. This book was written for you and because of you.

To my social butterfly wife, Barbara, who graciously dealt with me as I sat as a hermit in my small dark cave and created this amazing life giving program. Her input was valuable and provided more depth to the Living On High Speed network.

Acknowledgements

Thanks to my wife, Barbara, who edited and contributed to my first wellness guide. She walks the walk with me!

To my fellow Vita-Mix demonstrators, Ken Hiatt and Joe Tapper, who stand shoulder to shoulder with me to bring health to the masses via Vita-Mix raw food demonstrations.

To my friends who have joined the fight help the world become a healthier place and who provide support & encouragement while I continue to write, speak & educate: Pascal Cohen, Jean Pierre Petit, Lisa Lumiere, Illansy Ruiz, Penni Shelton, Markus Rothkranz, George Xavier Love, Fadi Moulouf, Jack Hays, Lee Sylvester, Jason Cirillo and many others!   Thank you for your work my friends.

To the health and wellness professionals who have shared their knowledge, who continue to lead the way and who are beacons of light. Personally, I send thanks to David Wolfe, Viktoras Kulvinskas, Lars Gustafsson and Brian Clement.

LIVING ON HIGH SPEED CONTENTS

Part 1

Life Is Change

Chapter 1

My Story Of Change

The first seventeen years of my life were a "bust", nutritionally speaking. My mother fed us well. But we consumed the typical Standard American Diet (SAD). We were a real "meat and potatoes" family. Our daily meals were comprised of meats such as pork and cheap hamburger being the mainstay. Most of our meals were accompanied by a starch, usually a potato in its many forms, fried, baked and boiled. And in a far place we occasionally consumed canned vegetables.

We thought we were eating healthy meals. But, I also recall eating many pre-processed / pre-packaged foods like white processed bread, spam, bologna, hot dogs, pizza, chicken pot pies, dumplings, pasta in its many forms such as macaroni and cheese, spaghetti and lasagna. We didn't think we were eating poorly. But the question is: Were we really thinking about good nutrition at all?

At the age of seventeen when I left home and joined the military, I made a decision to make mental, physical and even nutritional changes. Well, I thought so anyway. After all, I vowed to never eat hot dogs, bologna and pork products again. But, oddly enough I found myself cooking the same meals my mother had cooked. In-fact, I remember calling her on more than a few occasions to gain some of her old recipes.

My decision to join the military began a "change phase" in my adult life. This change phase I call a "purposed" change because I made a conscious decision. I decided at an early age to join the military and I intentionally set my goals to no longer eat the foods that were served in my home.

The next and most drastic change in my life came at the age of twenty. I remember it clearly. "Son, your mother is gone". I received this phone call from my father in the wee morning hours after Christmas Day. To say this was hard to hear is an understatement. Even though it was hard to hear, it was not a surprise. One year earlier my mother had fainted while working. An MRI revealed she had a brain tumor. The doctors did their best to remove the tumor but it was too far embedded into her brain. She was given a prognosis of six months if she underwent treatment. Yet, my Mom toughed it out for more than a year after receiving her prognosis date. Obviously I would call losing my mother at such a young age a "forced" change.

At the time of my Mother's cancer diagnosis, treatment and her death, I was stationed far away in the frozen tundra of Minot, North Dakota. I went home that year as often as I could to spend time with my dying mother and to help my family. But there never seemed to be enough time. With each successive visit I could see the damage that was being inflicted on her body and mind from the radiation and chemotherapy treatments. She lost her hair, became bloated, lost muscle mass and was constantly sick. Towards the end of her life my young mother could barely lift herself out of bed. The change she went through was frightening for my mother and family. This change was also confusing because we had no idea how to handle such adversity.

Was it the cancer directly that caused these drastic declines in my Mom's health? No it was not. The quick, drastic decline of her health was a direct result of the radiation, chemotherapy and other harsh chemicals that were administered to her body.

I once thanked the doctors who performed the operation to remove the tumor and cancer cells from her brain. I remember naively asking these questions "How did the cancer develop?" and "Why do you not eliminate cancer from her body with something other than those harsh life-altering chemicals?"

The doctor's answers forever impacted my life. They said, "Scott, we don't know exactly what caused this cancer and no other treatments exist to remove or cure cancer from the human body".

With all of the strength I could muster I asked these medical professionals; "If the body can *heal* itself from a cut or a broken limb, why can it not also heal itself of cancer?" The doctors gave me a flippant response that cancer is much more complicated than a mere cut or broken limb. Then they retreated to some inner office.

Their answer was unsatisfactory to me and fueled my drive to discover as much as I could about how human body heals itself. I first journeyed to the University of Maryland with the intent to become a better doctor in order to "prove them wrong". But I discovered that at that time mainstream medical training focused on disease *management* and had little to do with disease prevention or nurturing a true health & wellness lifestyle. At that time medical training did not incorporate instruction of stress management, deep nutritional therapy, proper breathing techniques, working out and other natural health concepts that have been proven to be effective. I did however learn that there was a mandatory eight hour nutrition class. Oh boy!

My observation was that most medical training was based mainly on disease diagnosis and management utilizing surgical and pharmaceutical methods.

This did not resonate well with me. Therefore, I decided to go in the opposite direction. I pursued a health & wellness focus and gained fitness certifications, nutrition certifications, EMT training and leadership training in order to help educate others.

I focused first on changing my own body. After successfully doing so, I trained many others to successfully improve their bodies. During my journey I morphed my body from 125 lbs to 185 lbs at five percent body fat within two years. As a bonus, I began to enjoy more physical adventures in life. I worked out, cliff dived, rock climbed, hiked, joined triathlon races, scuba dived, sky dived and many other fun and exciting things. This of course was a "purposed" change and a change that I enjoyed.

But two years later I experienced an unexpected "forced" change. A life altering skydiving accident occurred and left me for the worse. The details of this event are for another time. It is enough to say that I am thankful to be alive. But after the accident occurred I was left not being able to work-out or perform any of the "fun" physical activities. My physical rehabilitation persisted for years. As a result, within four years my muscles atrophied and my weight dropped from 185 lbs to 150 lbs. I became desk bound and to a small extent stopped enjoying life. When my military tour was near completion I decided against a third enlistment.

Then something occurred that happens to many of us. I experienced my first and so far only "unconscious" change. My downward spiral continued after my military separation and for more than two years I earned a very low income. My diet suffered as I ate cheap food during this phase. I learned the hard way that nutritious food is not cheap. The result of those two years was catastrophic. My body weight plummeted to 134 lbs and I became very sick. During this phase I experienced vertigo and a severe case of shingles.

I am not sure what to call the next change but I view it as a blessing. One of my good friends and a personal training client worked for a large telecom company. With his help I was able to obtain a management position within his company and I was finally able to eat more than *Ramen Noodles*. My corporate career flourished during this phase of my life but I found that I still could not physically workout. So, I poured my extra time and efforts into nutrition and wellness education.

What I learned during my studies was interesting. I observed that many well known and respected authorities of nutrition education referred to "living foods" and the benefits these foods provide.

I studied the works of educators such as Dr. Weil, Gary Null, Deepak Chopra, Eckhart Tolle, Hale Dwoskin, Penni Shelton, Brenda Cobb, Ann Wigmore, Dr. Ted Broer, Dr. Mercola, Markus Rothkranz, David Wolfe and many others. Their teachings were amazing and I respected their pursuit to empower the world to become healthier. I learned the benefits of eating more living foods and purposefully creating an energized life full of joy.

My most recent life change occurred roughly three years ago. This life change was the second most desired change in my family's life and we welcomed it with open arms. This change was a purposed change. We spent three years positioning ourselves to disconnect from the corporate machine and free ourselves from the "rat race". Our new journey as full time wellness consultants began. We also transitioned from "health-minded carnivores" to "life-loving", "living foods" enthusiast.

My journey has led me to understand that life is ever evolving and constantly changing. The many changes I have experienced have led me to a higher level of health and a path of higher energy living. I follow my passions and listen to my inner voice to guide my choices and experiences.

I now enjoy a life as an impassioned person who pursues his dreams and teaches others to do the same. I am a personal fitness trainer, Vita-Mix demonstrator, Certified Nutritionist, Certified David Wolfe Raw Food Nutritionist, Permaculture designer, blogger, author, seminar lecturer and a motivation and wellness coach.

I adhere to the following motto and in this book you will see why I do.

- Change Your Body
- Change Your Mind
- Change Your Energy
- Change Your Life

Chapter 2

Living On High Speed

So, if I could tell you what this book is about it would be this:

There are no magic pills and there is no one size fits all approach to improving your health. Acquiring true health is a journey and not a destination and to achieve total wellness one must utilize all aspects of wellness education. And most importantly life is about change. Some changes are forced on you, some are unconscious, some are mystical or spiritual and some changes you can create. Trust me when I say that it is no fun to have changes forced into your life. So I suggest before life forces a change on you and before an unconscious change occurs take the time to create the change you want in your life.

To this point I will teach you why it would be beneficial to:
- Live life with purpose.
- Eat living foods as often as possible.
- Include all aspects of wellness.
- Live life on high speed to attract higher energy.
- Use your high speed blenders.

We are what we eat or do not eat. We are what we live or do not live. We are what we do or do not do. We are who we associate with or do not associate with. We are what we plan and do not plan. We are what we live. So my question to you is: "Do you live your life on high speed?". Are you taking charge of your life or is your life taking charge of you? Your chance to change and improve your life is up to you and is now!

In this guide I will outline how "high speed blending", "high speed workouts", eating living foods and "living on high speed" have greatly improved hundreds of thousands of lives and might help you also. While this book was originally created for my high speed blender clients, I have since expanded it to also help any who are willing to regain their health through high speed blending, eating more live foods, focused high speed living, high speed workouts and much more.

I will explain why using these lifestyle tips will greatly improve your life making you feel more energized, alert, obtaining quicker fat loss, obtaining quicker muscle mass, better sleep, create greater success and much more.

And most importantly, I will share success steps with you from my life changing motto:

Change Your Body / Change Your Mind / Change Your Energy
to
Change Your Life

Part 2

The Heart Of Living On High Speed

Chapter 3

Intro To High Speed Blending (HSB)

Whole foods heal. Furthermore, research indicates that whole "live" foods contain hundreds if not thousands of powerful disease preventing nutrients, phyto-nutrients, enzymes, antioxidants and other yet to be discovered compounds. Additionally, it has been found that high speed blended whole foods have been shown to further help prevent chronic diseases such as cancer, diabetes, hypertension, heart disease and more.

One reason high speed blended foods are so healthy is because high speed machines such as Vita-Mix, BlendTec and Warring commercial machines have the ability to disrupt plant cell wall structure and significantly reduce food particle size which enhances the bioavailability of essential nutrients in fruits, vegetables and other plant based life. This particle size reduction includes all parts of the plant – skin, seeds, stems, leaves and the "meat" or fiber of the plant life. If blended long enough your whole food products can be reduced to a 95% particle reduction also known as bioavailability. Thus your digestive system will be able to easily absorb all of the life giving nutrients that your whole food provides.

Ruptured cell walls and superior particle reduction results in more released nutrients, increased absorbability and even better flavor.

Another benefit of high speed machines is their versatility. They perform the functions of at least 12 kitchen appliances.
1. Blender
2. Juice extractor
3. Food processor
4. Hot soup maker
5. Ice cream / Sorbet maker
6. Nut butter grinder
7. Grain mill
8. Mixer

9. Fondue maker
10. Milk processor- soy milk, almond milk, rice milk etc.
11. Coffee grinder
12. Meat grinder

Amazing high speed machines can perform these functions without ever changing one attachment. Life in the kitchen just became much more enjoyable and interesting.

In short, high speed blenders save you time & money, make the kitchen more enjoyable and they can drastically improve your health and lifestyle.

If you do not have a high speed blender, get one as soon as possible!

2hp or 3hp − What Option Is Better

What is true high speed? Many high speed blender manufactures advertise there is a significant difference in speed and / or nutritional results between a 2 hp or 3 hp machine. But is there?

Typically, high speed usually refers to machines in the commercial market place -bars, restaurants, smoothie / juice bars and health / wellness clinics. Thankfully, there are high speed devices available for residential use. Of these household models, the two most prominent brands are Vita-Mix and BlendTec. Now thanks in-part to slightly misguided marketing and sales campaigns, there seems to be a misconception in the marketplace that certain 3 hp machines perform better than 2 hp machines. For example, the Blendtec Connoisseur, Blendtec HP3A Blender, Total Blender, and even the Vita Mix Vita Prep 3 hp blenders all have a 3 hp motor and have been reported to be significantly more powerful than other machines such as the Vita-Mix 4500, 5000 and 5200. But the reality is that these 3 hp machines have been throttled down by a 13 or lower amp power supply. This means that their ceiling of applicable speed is similar to, albeit slightly faster than, a 2 hp blender.

But the good news is that research has proven that 2 hp machines perform equally well in breaking down the cellular wall of fruits, vegetables and plants. 2

hp machines simply take one to two minutes longer to do the job. But they do get the job done.

High speed machines with 2 hp or 3 hp that use lower amp settings are sufficient for residential use and are less expensive. Lower amp machines can produce the same food product as a 3 hp and higher amp blenders but just require a little longer spin time. Keep in mind that additional spinning equates to more processing and more heat. Be careful not to over-process or over-heat your "living food". Therefore, I recommend purchasing a 15 or higher amp machine. Both Vita-Mix and Blendtec offer these higher amp options.

Juicing vs. High Speed Blending

High Speed Blending Facts

It's about the fiber!
- Fiber fills you.
- Fiber stabilizes and controls your blood sugar levels.
- Fiber carries as much as 86% of the nutrient profile of your fruits and vegetables.
- Fiber cleanses your body and keeps you regular.

Consider this, when you purchase your fresh produce you pay by the pound. Yet when you use a juice extractor, the meat of your produce (otherwise known as fiber) is separated and discarded. Thus you are wasting 50% to 75% of your money.

In addition to the waste debate, there is a considerable amount of controversy between juicing or blending foods. Both juicing and high speed blending unlock vital nutrients from foods. Personally I highly recommend owning both a high speed blender and a juicer (either a press or masticator).

These machines can be quite expensive, but I believe both are an essential part of any raw, vegan, & health enthusiast's kitchen. So be sure to start a "saving up" for your future health.

Did you know that most of the nutrients of plants, fruits and vegetables are stored in the cell walls? Fortunately most fruits and vegetables can be well absorbed by your digestive system if you chew your food adequately. But let's face it. For the most part, we are a nation of "fast food and fast lifestyle fanatics". This means we usually only take a few small bites and then swallow. This is of course very hard on your digestive system. But the good news is that if you take the time to chew thoroughly then you can process your food down to a 70% to 75% absorbability rate.

That being stated, I must tell you that there are a few plants like kale, seaweed and herbs that are extremely tough and almost impossible to fully masticate even if you chew for a long time. High speed blenders excel here. When produce is blended in a high speed blender particle reduction produces as great as 95% absorbability. This improved particle reduction ensures that the cell walls of your produce, plants, stems, leaves, seeds, seaweeds, weeds, and other tough plants have been ruptured. Ruptured cell walls mean more released nutrients, more flavor and greater absorbability.

Be aware that high speed blender blades move at such extreme high speeds that heat is generated through friction. At temperatures above 115 degrees, a plant's natural enzymes will become denatured. Thus your food is no longer considered "live" or "raw". The easy fix to keeping your enzymes intact and active is to maintain a lower temperature. Therefore, add something cool like ice or frozen fruits/vegetables while blending. Or simply do not spin your produce long enough to create high temperatures. By the way, it usually takes at least 3, 4 or maybe even 5 minutes of high speed blending to reach 115 degrees depending on the initial temperature of the liquid base.

Juicing Facts

Fiber rich juicing is one of the best features of your high speed blender (HSB). Juicing "rules" vary slightly with HSBs so keep the following explanation in mind. When you place 4 apples into your HSB and spin on high for 30 to 40 seconds, the result is applesauce not apple juice. The apple has a high fiber to liquid ratio. To create apple juice, add liquid in the form of purified water or juice or ice.

HSBs do a great job at emulsifying. For our purposes in nutrition, the HSB are capable of making an emulsion. By definition, an emulsion is "a suspension of small globules of one liquid in a second liquid with which the first will not mix, such as milk fats in milk". Therefore, using a HSB allows one to drink the fiber of the apple in an apple juice. Fiber-rich juices contain as much as 80% more nutrient value than extracted juice. And yes a HSB can reduce the fiber so fine as to ensure there is no "pulp" or grit in your juice, considering the appropriate amount of spin time is used. This type of processing creates a bioavailability rating between 90 to 95 percent of your juices, soups and purees.

Are you looking for an absorbability rate even greater than 95%? Rejoice! There is a way to achieve 100% absorbability using your HSB. Simply filter the emulsified liquid (juice, milk or soup) using a cheese cloth or nut-milk bag. Only very fine, undetectable particles of fiber will remain in your liquid and your digestive system will absorb it completely.

If you still prefer using a " juice extractor", I recommend either a slow turning, masticating-type of juicer or a press- style juicer like the Norwalk. I believe that the Norwalk juicer is the best juice extractor on the planet because absolutely none of the liquid juice is wasted. The extracted fiber is so dry that it is probably flammable. An additional benefit of the Norwalk is easier clean up.

I do not recommend using a juice extractor for long periods of time. Juice extracting is best for detoxing and cleansing your body and having an occasional delicious drink.
Juice that is extracted has dense nutrients, concentrated sugar and no fiber. Although the drink tastes delicious, there is no fiber to slow down the absorption of sugar into your bloodstream. There exists the opportunity for blood sugar fluctuations.

Now don't get me wrong. Juicing has done many people well. But the human body is designed to digest food. The digestive process actually begins in the mouth with chewing the food. Chewing stimulates saliva production and enzymes. Long term juicing / fluid diets alter this system and can lead to changes in digestive enzymes, stomach acid levels, bowel movements, flora bacteria populations and other digestive issues.

Another drawback to juice extractors compared to HSB is the time required for clean up. Extra cleaning is required to remove fiber from the extractor wheel and / or sieve or strainer basket.

Additionally, centrifugal-type extractors leave valuable, nutritious liquid in the pulp which is discarded. To regain this lost juice, squeeze the pulp through a nut- milk bag. Let it hang over a cup or pitcher and in about 10 minutes you can capture more juice from the fiber.

Again, pure juicing in my opinion is reserved for detoxing, cleansing, disease management and an occasional delicious drink. Pure "fiber-less" juice is absorbed quickly and directly into your bloodstream. This puts minimal pressure on your digestive system. For a limited time and for disease management this is fine.

Did you know that vegetable juice is typically much healthier for you and contains less concentrated sugar than fruit juice? However, fruit juicing has healthy benefits also.

Typically fruits have more antioxidants and different phytonutrients than vegetables. So add to your diet fruits and fruit juices occasionally. Primarily stick with veggie juicing for detoxing and cleansing your body. Also realize that extended fruit juicing places strain on your pancreas, kidneys and other parts of your body because the high sugar content creates excess insulin. And in some cases like bacteria over growth, Candida, cancer, yeast overgrowth and sugar management issues, it may be necessary to avoid all sugars (for a short time) even sugar from fruit.

For best healing results drink a vegetable juice on an empty stomach first in the morning. Wait 20 minutes before consuming anything else. This timing allows for the proper absorption of the juice and the nutrients in the juice into your digestive tract.

There are volumes written on the subject of juice extracting so doing a little of your own research will likely ensure greater success and happiness.

Blendtec / Vitamix Comparison

Over the years I have been repeatedly asked which HSB machine is best, Blendtec or Vitamix? The reality is that both machines ROCK. High speed blenders perform functions that no other one kitchen appliance can. Both are well worth your investment. That being stated, I have placed a few comparisons below to help you better understand the differences. In the end, I recommend you purchase either machine and get started Living On High Speed.

Automated vs. Manual Control

VitaMix

Vitamix machines offer complete manual control of your blending process (except for a few specific commercial models). Vitamix uses switch technology which includes a variable speed dial and a Hi/Lo switch. These machines also come with a tamper to assist in blending solid and whole (uncut) foods. The tamper is not needed for all meals but is extremely helpful when making frozen desserts, nut butters and thick recipes like hummus.

The manual nature of these machines allows for customized blending times to allow your recipes to reach your preferred texture.

As of the completion of this book VitaMix has released an automated machine. This new addition to the family is called the Pro 500. This machine combines the manual switch technology with three new automated pre-programmed timing cycles.

Blendtec

Blendtec machines offer automated control of your blending process. Blendtec uses push button technology along with pre-programmed cycles that allow you to push a button and walk away during the blending process. While automated cycles can be helpful, some recipes require the blending process to be restarted because the pre-programmed cycle often ends before the food particles have been fully blended to your satisfaction. This is not the case with most of the meals but it does occur when harder elements like carrots and beets or whole fruits like apples or frozen material like whole frozen strawberries are added to the container. Blendtec does offer manual control on a few models which interestingly eliminates the need for the automated blending cycles. But please note that to use the manual control, you must hold down the button during the manual process.

Blendtec suggests that a tamper is never needed when using their machines. But I have found that there are times when a tamper is needed even when using a Blendtec machine, especially when creating a smooth ice cream or when placing whole items like carrots and apples into the machine.

The manual nature of the Vitamix is more widely accepted and more often used by health clinics, bars and restaurants because the manual nature ensures a smoother and more bio-available meal.

Blendtec and Vitamix both easily crush ice, make hot soups, nut butters, grind seeds, puree fruit, make smoothies, grind refined flour and a whole lot more. Both machines excel at breaking down the celluar walls of the plant life. Though the VitaMix draws less power at *11.5 amps/1380 watts* versus the Blendtec's *13 amps/1560 watts*, I have found that the Vitamix can blend anything that the Blendtec can and in some cases can make things much more smooth and creamy.

If you are looking for more power than the standard consumer machines then please know that both Vita-Mix and Blendtec offer 3hp machines that have higher amp ratings including 15 and even 20 amp machines. Vita-Mix now even offers a 4hp machine. But these commercial options are a higher price point and not necessary to achieve the 95% bioavailability.

Both blenders are noisy because of their high speed but the Blendtec is noticeably louder.

Smoothie / Juice Making

Both the Vitamix and the Blendtec excel at making amazing smoothies and juices.

But as mentioned previously in order to create super smooth green smoothies in the Blendtec one will sometimes need to re-run the cycle or use the manual button. This may occur rarely.

It was found that creamy and super smooth green smoothies can be created consistently using the Vitamix regardless of the quantity of greens that are packed into the container.

In regards to juicing, remember the basic juicing guides that were discussed earlier. Add the proper amount of liquid to your container and either machine will break down the cell walls of your plants reducing the particle size from 90% to 95% bioavailability. What happens next is very cool. It is called emulsification. In short, the machines combine the liquid with the fiber making an awesome fiber- rich juice. But again if you want a truly "pulp" free drink then remove the remaining pulp by using a cheesecloth or a nut milk bag. What is left is still a fiber- rich juice that is healthier for you than standard juice which has no fiber.

Using The Machines as Grain Mills

Blendtec advertises "one blade does it all" and claims that Vita-Mix is inferior because it requires two different blades; wet-blade & dry blade. Interestingly, Blendtec sells an attachment called the Kitchen Mill.

In reality, identical flour consistency results from grains milled in the Vitamix "wet blade" and from the standard Blendtec container. I call this"heavy" flour. It is refined enough to make bread and cake batter.

Flours resulting from grains milled in the Vita-Mix dry blade or the Blendtec Kitchen Mill are comparable. The flour is much finer. I call this a "light" flour which is refined enough to make "flaky" pastry dough. These blades are also better at grinding herbs and spices.

Warranty and Durability

Vitamix has the Commercial HSB industry's best warranty: A complete 7 year full use warranty. The Blendtec offers a limited 3 years warranty. Both the Blendtec and Vitamix are well known for great customer service honoring their warranties without hassle. Both offer extended warranty services.

Longevity and reliability has made the Vitamix machine the #1 rated blender in the commercial marketplace. Over 89,000 professional bars, restaurants and smoothie houses use Vitamix. Vitamix provides an average of 25 years of reliable, residential usage. However, some customers have enjoyed over 50 years of service.

My comparison summary is simple. Both machines are great but the Vitamix is superior because it outlasts all competition.

Part 3

You Are What You Eat

Chapter 4

There's Life In The Food You Eat

We all have heard "You are what you eat". But do we believe it? Or do we stop to think about it? I dare say NO. If we did, then I imagine that our nation would not be 66% overweight, obese and disease bound.

Your body contains roughly 60 trillion cells all of which work in balance to keep you healthy. But seven years from now not one of those cells will be the same cell that resides inside of you today. Daily a metabolic process called hyperplasia occurs. This process is the act of the old cell splitting and dividing to create new cells. This occurs because your cells work 24/7 on your behalf. These busy cells lose steam and the ability to keep you healthy so they send in reinforcements.

These cells require ample amounts of the key nutrients to maintain this busy schedule. Yet most Americans consume what is called the SAD diet (Standard American Diet). This SAD diet is composed mainly of processed foods, fast foods, high fat and high caloric but low nutrient dense foods.

So, what do you think is rebuilding your cells; magic, the thin air, or the SAD items you place into your body? Yep you guessed correctly. The items that you ingest on a daily basis are actually re-building your body. Seven years from now you could be a processed "Twinkie" or a "Nutrient dense disease fighting machine that is filled with life'. I trust you will choose life.

Additionally, not only are we a direct result of "what we eat", but also "how we eat"! Many factors such as the time intervals in which we eat, stress levels, and how we eat should also be considered. We should realize the dramatic effects on the human metabolism when either meals are skipped or when stomachs are gorged. Eating smaller meals more frequently throughout the day contributes to a healthier metabolism.

Again, as a reminder most people do not properly chew their food. In a perfect world, food should be chewed over 30 times before swallowing. This allows for easier digestion. But then again, it is not a perfect world. Therefore, your HSB can save the day by doing the chewing for you!

Living vs. Cooked Foods

Maybe you are asking "What are living foods?" Living foods are any plant based foods that have recently been harvested from the Earth and have not been heated above 115 degrees.

In some cases, these plants can be dried and dehydrated at low temperatures and are still considered "live" by many health enthusiast. I personally prefer foods that have not been dried and I try to stick to local plants recently harvested from their growth source. The closer the food source is to you, the later it can be harvested and the more viable nutrients that will be inside of your plant based foods.

The plant kingdom has many awesome elements that are beneficial to the human body; minerals, vitamins, phytonutrients, enzymes and even a "life force". All of these elements, specifically the enzymes in live food, have a heat intolerance factor. When heated beyond their tolerance levels, enzymes denature or become weak and are unable to effectively metabolize plant nutrients.

Eating live foods or "going raw" seems to be a new trend. In reality however, humans have been eating live foods aka "raw" foods since the dawn of time. Unfortunately, since the industrial revolution more and more processed and pre-packaged convenient fast foods have replaced living fresh foods. But the good news is that there seems to be a resurgence of Living Plants / Raw and Vegan awareness.

There is also a "life force" to all living things. Although still being researched, I am sure the life force begins to decline after the plant is harvested from the source. Therefore eating fruits and vegetables as close to harvest as possible is the best option and the most beneficial to your health and to your taste buds.

Additionally, research has shown us that boiling water changes its molecular structure. There are indications that the human body produces white blood cells to attack over-heated foods as an infection while "live" plants do not cause a rise in your white blood count. Thus it would appear that "live" food is accepted as a "friend" to your body.

Is a "raw" or "vegan" diet the only way to improve your health? The answer of course is "no". Over the last few decades hundreds of diet types have been created and have helped millions of people become healthy and fit.

But out of all of the diet types in the world, there is only one that I and thousands of other nutrition experts recommend when trying to combat major diseases such as cancer, rare blood disorders, fibromyalgia and many other difficult disorders. And that diet is a diet based on eating live plants. The live and raw plant kingdom has every element needed to keep you healthy and to combat disease.

So the moral of the story is: If you want to stay as healthy as possible for as long as possible then eat uncooked plant based foods that are local as often as possible.

Does this mean you need to consume "live" foods 100% of the time? No it does not. But, I recommend consuming "live" foods as often as possible. Try at least 70% to 80% and I know you will feel an increase in your energy in a very short time. If your goal is a 100% living foods diet then go about the change slowly and intuitively. Meaning, listen to your body and do not push it too far, too fast.

Do you think this is impossible or not fun? Think again! Tens of millions of people have made the transition to a living foods diet and are enjoying life.

Lastly, there are two types of Raw / Living Food methods.

1. Living Foods – Simplified (LFS)
    a. This is the method I follow. With this method living food enthusiasts enjoy their live foods as close and direct from the vine as possible. LFS individuals typically lead busy lives and do not like spending too much time in the kitchen prepping food. They eat fresh fruits, vegetables, herbs and wild plants by hand, in salad form or in blended form and rarely use their time to dehydrate or

create foods like crackers, raw breads, raw cookies, raw cakes and etc.

2. Living Foods – Gourmet (LFG)
    a. This is the method my wife loves to follow (I of course do all of the prep work for her.). With this method LFG individuals love gourmet foods regardless if they lead busy lives. They want cakes, cookies, bread, cheese (non-dairy of course), and a host of other prepared foods. Basically they want the "old" lifestyle they used to enjoy but made with better living ingredients. They want "to have their cake and eat it too".
    b. Delicious gourmet recipes are possible in the raw food world. One just needs to spend a little more time in the kitchen dehydrating, sprouting, making non dairy cheeses, sauces and other time consuming delicious recipes.

Either method is acceptable and highly enjoyable. I recommend trying both.

In summary; purchase local produce, pick local wild weeds that are nutritious and stay away from store produce that is shipped long distances or from other countries. And of course don't overheat your food. Your body will love you for it and reward you with higher energy. And you will love your body!

To Be Organic Or Not To Be Organic

That is the question. Well it is not so much a question of should you enjoy organics as it is a question of affordability, availability and believability. Unfortunately organic products are more expensive thus could cause a challenge for some. But with some research one may be able to find very affordable organics.

Since organic food has become popular there are big retail health stores that have also grown popular. But instead of going big, go small. Get in contact with your local farmers and try to purchase directly. Search out local farmers markets and shop at local small fresh food markets. These local stores can offer a host of surprises. They often have fresher produce, friendlier people, lower prices and even support local farmers. I have even found great prices and organic produce at oriental markets. Certain hard to find products can be ordered via the internet.

If one has no choice or options to go organic then I have a few tips to help you eat somewhat clean while consuming conventional foods. For instance, focus on removing from your diet those foods that carry the heaviest burden of pesticides, additives and hormones. According to the USDA Environmental Working Group (EWG), consumers can reduce their pesticide exposure by 80% by avoiding the most contaminated fruits and vegetables and eating only the cleanest. If consumers get their USDA-recommended 5 daily servings of fruits and veggies from the 15 most contaminated, they could consume a minimum of 10 pesticides a day. Those who eat the 15 least contaminated conventionally grown produce ingest less than 2 pesticides daily.

Since 1995 the EWG has been publishing a guide called the "Dirty Dozen" highlighting the most pesticide contaminated foods. The dirty dozen list only reflects measurable pesticide residues on the parts of the foods normally consumed (i.e. after being washed and peeled). These 12 foods are listed below.

The Dirty Dozen

Fruits and vegetables are an essential part of a healthy diet. But many conventional varieties contain pesticide residues that are embedded into the fruit/veggie meat and therefore cannot be removed by washing the surface.

Government testing shows that you can reduce your exposure to pesticides by as much as 80% if you avoid the most contaminated foods in the grocery store.

Again the best way to avoid ingesting pesticide residue is to purchase organic produce. The other option is to be clear on which conventional produce retain pesticides and other dangerous residue after being washed. This list is called the "Dirty Dozen". The Dirty Dozen was created in 1995 by a USDA department titled the Environmental Working Group (EWG). The Dirty Dozen list is updated annually.

2010 Dirty Dozen:
Celery

Peaches
Strawberries
Apples
Blueberries
Nectarines
Bell peppers
Spinach
Kale
Cherries
Potatoes
Grapes

The Clean 15

Not all non-organic fruits and vegetables have a high pesticide level after being washed. Some produce has a strong outer layer that provides a defense against pesticide contamination. The EWG also found a number of non-organic fruits and vegetables dubbed as the "Clean 15" that retained little to no pesticides after being washed.

2010 Clean 15:
Onions
Avocados
Sweet corn
Pineapples
Mango
Sweet peas
Asparagus
Kiwi fruit
Cabbage
Eggplant
Cantaloupe
Watermelon
Grapefruit
Sweet potatoes
Sweet onions

Chapter 5

Top Foods To Avoid / Top Foods To Eat

So many diets so much confusion: Adkins, Eat Right 4 Your Blood Type, Zone, Raw, Vegan, Vegetarian, Fit For Life, South Beach, Cookie Diet, Jenny Craig, Eat For Health, Hallelujah Diet, Kosher and numerous other religious diets. The list goes on and on. In fact, there are now well over 568 documented diet programs on the market and more popping up every day.

Which if any of these diets work? Well, to some degree all of them do, at least some of the time. Because most of these programs do seem to work for many people, there has been some confusion and some massive exaggerations as to which program is the best. So the question is: Is there a best?

Sometimes there is a "best" for you. It all depends on your body type, the state of your body and much more. While amazing results can be achieved from each of these programs, many individuals have not achieved their desired results while others have.

Here are just a few of the reasons some if not all of these diet programs do not always work for everyone.

- **Cheating** – Many people believe they are adhering to the program but not everyone sticks to any one program 100% of the time. Cheating even just a small amount makes it impossible to judge the efficiency of any particular program. The best way to stay on track is to keep an accurate food and workout log.
- **Quitting** – We are a society of fast food and fast lifestyle people and we expect things to come easy. Attaining great health does not come easily or accidently. Great health is achieved with consistency.
- **Plateau** – Some people are not aware they have hit the plateau or are not sure how to correct such a problem. This is very common and can be reversed if you consistently apply changes to your program or occasionally switch to a new program. This way your body will constantly make changes to keep up with you.

- **Clogged Intestines** - Your colon needs to be cleansed. If you have been eating the SAD diet, then you need to be cleansed and detoxified. PERIOD

- **One Size Does Not Fit All** – Not every program is for every "body". Each person's body chemistry is different. This often creates the need for a different program for many people.

- **Weak Stomach Acid** – Part of a balanced pH. system includes a strong stomach acid level. Weak stomach acid results in un-dissolved and under digested foods. Your digestive system relies on your food particles being totally dissolved for proper absorption.

- **Critters Are Eating Your Food** – Yup I said it. A diet rich in processed foods and animal products is a diet rich in parasites and parasitical foods. And if you remember your biology, just a few parasite eggs can and will quickly multiply into millions of hungry parasites. And believe me, all humans have parasites. Even if you don't or have not eaten meat it is possible to acquire parasites from the ground, the air, and many objects you touch. These parasites eat the food you ingest robbing you of the life giving nutrients that your foods should be providing you. Parasites left untreated prevent proper weight loss, damage vital organs and muscle and cause many diseases. Detox your body and cleanse it regularly!

- **Food Combining Problems** – Each food type fruit, vegetables, meat, dairy, water, bread and etc. require different levels of time to become fully dissolved and absorbed by the digestive tract. When combining these different food types a fermentation process could begin which can cause bloating, clogging and other digestion related issues.

- **Your Body Is Toxic** – A toxic body cannot flush nutrients through its system properly. Heavy metals, drugs (pharmaceutical and non pharma), household cleaners, skin and body care products and a host of other pollutants get trapped your body and keep you from attaining optimum health. Yet another reason to detox and cleanse your body.

- **Low Enzymes** – Enzymes are the key elements in breaking down food. Natural living plants, fruits and vegetables contain enzymes. Yet most of us do not consume the proper amount of live active enzymes required to properly metabolize all foods. Your body does create enzymes. But, if your system is compromised then sufficient enzyme levels cannot be generated.

- **Sleep / Rest / Meditation / Stress** – Stress of all types wreaks havoc on the body. In specific, cortisol is released when the body is not rested, relaxed and peaceful. Get your sleep, train your mind and body to relax and de-stress yourself.
- **Genetics** – Yes genetics play a role in your health. But do not use genetics as an excuse. Research has proven that normal DNA can be altered. Likewise, bad or damaged DNA can be corrected!! Plus "bad" DNA typically only constitutes about 15% of the factors preventing your best health.

Don't let one of these "road blocks" block you from becoming your best!

The Top Foods to Avoid

If living foods provide life and cooked foods bring harm then is it possible that processed "dead" food brings death?

I would suggest yes. Today's processed foods are loaded with sugars, salts and fats to make them taste good. But more importantly processed foods contain chemical additives that are considered to be toxic to the body. These chemicals are typically inserted into foods to preserve the shelf life, enhance the smells and enhance the taste of your foods. Processed foods may not be a "strong" poison that kills instantly but they poison slowly. Because your body does not recognize these chemicals as food, they are not digested but stored in various organs, body fat, soft tissue, glands and even your blood.

Most chemicals are very difficult to eliminate from the body. Deep cleanse programs often miss certain heavy metals and other hard to reach chemical storage areas.

So, what is the point? ***Don't Eat Processed Foods***

Processed foods do not provide life giving nutrients and are in most cases considered to be dangerous for your body. All processed foods should be avoided but focusing on removing the worst or most deadly foods from your diet should be your first priority.

Additionally, as you remove from your diet the foods listed below and add more living foods, you will find that more energy and life will be given back to your body.

1. Pork, high fat luncheon meats, ham, pepperoni, hot dogs, bacon and sausage meat.
2. Shellfish: oysters, scallops, clams, crab and lobster. They are scavengers and feed off the bottom of the ocean. Also contain high levels of mercury.
3. Aspartame: Nutrasweet, Equal and most other artificial sweeteners.
4. Hydrogenated, partially hydrogenated oils or lard.
5. Junk Food: snack cakes, candy, cola, fast food, pizza etc.
6. Dairy products: milk, cheese, creams, yogurts and other bovine produced milk elements.
7. Chlorinated water. Chlorine is a deadly toxin. "Either use a filter or become a filter"!
8. Alcohol: Just 1 oz of alcohol reduces the body's ability to burn fat by 30%.
9. Pasta & Breads: the only breads I recommend are sprouted grain products like Ezekiel.
10. And the last but one of the most important items to remove from your diet is all **fried food**! Heated and superheated oil is DANGEROUS. Research shows us that oils, when heated, degrade easily into toxic compounds and release dangerous free radicals. Prolonged consumption of burnt oils lead to atherosclerosis, inflammatory joint disease, development of birth defects and a host of other inflammatory diseases.

Top Foods To Blend

There are many foods and many recipes to be enjoyed and prepared in your HSB. There is rarely a "wrong" answer. Usually it is a matter of taste.

To help get you started I have created a guide (see below) that answers the question: What are the "top" foods I should add to my HSB?

The following chart contains the highest nutrient dense- foods (superfoods not included) as rated by Dr. Joel Fuhrman who created the "Aggregate Nutrient Density Index" (ANDI).

An ANDI score indicates the nutrient density of a food on a scale from 1 to 1000. ANDI scores are calculated by evaluating a range of micronutrients including vitamins, minerals, phytochemicals and antioxidant capacities. The higher the concentration of these elements in a food per calorie the higher its ANDI score. Kale, for instance, is a dark leafy green which scores 1000 while soda has a score of 1.

Using The Quick Reference Chart - Chose 1 item from the Greens column and 1 or 2 items from the Fruit column and 1 item from the Liquid column and feel free to add optional items like Protein and Superfoods to create a complete nutritious and delicious meal. Within 45 to 70 seconds you will have the most nutrient dense smoothie / juice around.

Quick Reference High Nutrient Density Chart

PS_BX03427297

CreateSpace
7290 Investment Drive Suite B
North Charleston, SC 29418

3/07/2014 01:12:45 AM
rder ID: 58871837

ty.	Item
	IN THIS SHIPMENT
	Living On High Speed
	1463618336

Greens	Fruit	Liquid	Optional Protein	Optional Super Foods
½ Cup Mustard Greens	1 Cup Strawberries	Young Coconut Water	Spirulina	Any from Chapter 6
1 Cup Watercress	1 Cup Pomegranate Juice	Fresh Vegetable Juice	Chlorella	Any from Chapter 6
1 Cup Kale	2 Plums	Fresh Celery Juice	Bee Pollen	Any from Chapter 6
½ Cup Turnip Greens	1 Cup Raspberries	Fresh Fruit Juice	Hemp Seeds	Any from Chapter 6
Collard Greens	1 Cup Blueberries	Pure Alkaline Water	Chia Seeds	Any from Chapter 6
2 Cup Spinach	½ Grapefruit	Pure Ice	Protein Powders	Any from Chapter 6
2 Cup Bok Choy	1 Orange		Pea, soy, whey	Any from Chapter 6
1 Cup Brussel Sprouts	1 Cup Cantaloupe			
	1 Kiwi			
	1 Cup Watermelon			
	½ Apple			
	1 Peach			

Add a "Daily Basic" Nutrient To Create A Perfect Meal!

Less Liquid To Thicken, More Liquid To Thin

To alkalize add: pinch sea salt, 1/8 tsp baking soda & 8 drops trace minerals

TIP - Avoid sugar of all types (including fruit) while dealing with issues such as bacteria overgrowth, Candida, yeast problems, cancer and other sugar feeding diseases.

Chapter 6

The Super Foods

The term **"Superfood"** is often misused, over-used or even misunderstood by many people. But generally most experts do agree that there are certain foods that are low caloric / high nutrient foods. Superfoods typically contain superior sources of anti-oxidants, phytonutrients, vitamins, minerals and other essential life giving nutrients that other foods do not.

Superfoods can be found in various forms and locations. Unfortunately, most cannot be found in your local grocery stores or even farmers markets.

I have listed below a few of the top superfoods that I recommend and use myself. Each of these can be added to any one of your blended recipes. Some add a great taste and others not so much. But all add awesome amounts of life giving nutrients to help nourish and heal your body.

You can go to www.livingonhighspeed.com to discover how to obtain super foods that I use.

The Daily Basics

The "Daily Basics" are just a few food items that I consider should be part of your high speed meals on a daily basis.

Enzymes – Many nutrition experts call enzymes the "spark" of life because they play a necessary role in virtually all of the biochemical activities that occur in the body. They are essential for digesting food, for metabolizing nutrients, for stimulating the brain, for providing cellular energy and for repairing tissues, organs and cells.

The functions of enzymes are so many and so diverse that it would be impossible to list all. But the easiest designation is that enzymes are often divided into two main groups: digestive enzymes and metabolic enzymes.

Digestive enzymes will be the focus for this discussion.

Digestive enzymes breakdown the foods you eat. They metabolize the nutrients like vitamins, minerals, phytochemicals enabling them so they can be absorbed into the bloodstream for use in multiple bodily functions.

While the body does manufacture a supply of enzymes, it can and does also obtain enzymes from the fruits and vegetables you eat. Unfortunately enzymes are sensitive to heat and most will denature at temperatures greater than 115 degrees. Therefore, maintaining a temperature below 115 degrees, or consuming raw foods yields the highest and most benefit from the enzymes.

Also taking enzyme supplements before every cooked meal will greatly improve your nutritional absorption rate of cooked foods. And taking enzymes after a raw meal will greatly improve your absorption rate of living foods.

For the best benefit, any enzyme supplements you chose should contain all of the major enzyme groups to include amylase, protease and lipase.

For even better digestion also use the following items on an as-needed basis: apple cider vinegar, HCl pills to quickly strengthen weak stomach acid, Celtic sea salt and at night take probiotics.

Probiotics – In a healthy state, the body has a higher concentration of good bacteria than bad, or disease-causing, bacteria.

But most of us do not live in a healthy state. Instead the human body has become full of bacteria-destroying elements called antibiotics. Antibiotics kill both good and bad bacteria alike. These nasty little things are in many of the foods you eat; milk, fish, meat and anything else that big farms raised. Animals that are raised in crowded conditions and live in close proximity to each other, contract and share diseases with each other. To combat sickness, farmers administer massive amounts of antibiotics to livestock. When meat or milk products are consumed, these antibiotics persist and are transferred to you. These antibiotics deplete your bacteria levels and drain your immune system leaving you vulnerable to infection.

Research on probiotics is fascinating. In short, probiotics are the best line of defense your body has to defend itself from infection. Most people do not realize it but the "gut" carries as much as 70% of your immune system. And in your gut sits millions if not billions of bacteria. These bacteria keep us healthy and aid in many other functions. Probiotics are good bacteria and should remain in high levels in your gut. I recommend consuming natural and supplemental probiotics on a daily basis!

Good bacteria can be obtained through two sources. The first is direct from the Earth. As children, we play in the dirt and bacteria invades the body. Yes, some of the bacteria sources are harmful but much of the soil based bacteria is beneficial. But in this clean world of antiviral soaps and cleaners and most of us no longer working outdoors I fear we have lost touch with nature. This departure from nature, coupled with the bacteria killing cleaners moves us farther and farther away from good bacteria and good health.

The second way to obtain good bacteria is to purchase probiotic supplements. There are many on the market. Look for the highest probiotic count possible when purchasing these supplements. Probiotics that utilize "soil based organisms" are better and stronger.

I suggest you ingest ample amounts of probiotics every day and go outside every now and again and walk barefoot through the dirt and grass (watch out for the dog poo). You will be much happier and healthier for it.

Essential Fatty Acids – All fats are not created equally. PERIOD. Essential Fatty Acids (EFA's) are fats that the body cannot produce on its own and are available through one of two sources: 1) Plant sources like Flax, Borage, Primrose, Hemp, Chia and other plants. 2) Fish, specifically deep sea fish like mackerel, salmon and krill.

EFAs remain liquid at room temp and stay liquid in your body. EFA's help tremendously with many bodily functions such as, but certainly not limited to, hair growth, digestion, cell repair, cell detoxing, skin repair and growth, proper brain functions, stabilizing blood sugar levels, keeping proper HDL/LDL levels in balance and much more!

The primary function of essential fats is to coat and protect your cell walls. Your cell walls are susceptible to damage without this protective barrier.

I recommend that you put a little research into this subject and you will be the better for it. I highlight a few other facts about EFA's later in the book but please note that this is yet another substance the body requires daily.

Green leafy vegetables - Green leafy vegetables are the rock stars of the plant kingdom. They are highly nutritious and readily available. But if you are American then you probably do not eat enough of them. Now I must admit that if you are one of the many faithful high speed blender enthusiasts, you probably consume more leafy greens than the average American.

Fresh, raw, green, leafy vegetables contain high doses of chlorophyll, easily digestible proteins, enzymes and a wide range of phytonutrients, vitamins and minerals. These particular vegetables also act as a health tonic for the brain and immune system and a cleanser of the kidneys.

Leafy greens are denser in nutrients than other vegetables and contain awesome amounts of calcium.

Leafy greens should definitely be a large part of your daily diet!

Green Superfoods

Leafy green vegetables are not the only green things that are good for us. Superfoods come in green. They have higher concentrations of easily digestible nutrients, phytonutrients, fiber and vitamins and minerals to protect and heal the body. They also contain many beneficial substances such as proteins, protective phyto-chemicals and healthy bacteria which builds cleaner muscles and tissues, aid digestive functions and more effectively protect you against disease and illness.

Green superfoods are extremely rich in chlorophyll. Chlorophyll greatly increases the production of hemoglobin in the bloodstream. Oxygen-rich blood is the first and most important element for cells to thrive and stay healthy.

Wheat Grass - Wheatgrass juice is considered by many people to be one of the healthiest drinks. It is the sprouted grass of a wheat seed. It should be harvested before the wheat kernel forms. Because it is not developed into a whole grain it does not contain gluten or other common allergic agents. Wheat grass is super alkalizing and is excellent for promoting healthy blood. It helps combat high blood pressure, diabetes, gastritis, ulcers, liver disease, asthma, eczema, hemorrhoids, skin infections, anemia, constipation, body odor, bleeding gums, burns, even cancer.

Grasses and other leafy greens have a tough cellulose structure. To get their benefit we must "juice or blend them". Most people "juice" wheat grass using a specialized leafy greens juice extractor. But it is also feasible to throw a handful in your high speed blender. Thus, once again, you will receive the fiber and all of the benefits of the nutrient dense water inside of the grass. Plus in blended form, wheat grass loses its strong grassy taste of the highly concentrated juice. Wheat grass is easy to grow indoors and outdoors.

Barley Grass – Barley grass is similar to wheat grass in nutrient density but also high in calcium, iron, bio-flavonoids and Vitamin B12 which is very important in a vegetarian diet. It is also host anti-viral properties and is known to heal stomach, duodenal, pancreatitis and colon disorders.

Blue Green Algae – Blue green algae contains virtually every nutrient. It has a 60% protein content and a more complete amino acid profile than beef. It contains one of the best known food sources of beta carotene, B vitamins and chlorophyll. It has been shown to improve brain function and memory, strengthen the immune system and help with viruses, colds and flu.

Spirulina - Spirulina is another algae source and is one of the highest known protein sources on Earth containing 70% complete absorbable protein. Spirulina is recognized throughout the world as the most promising of all algae as it is considered to be an immediately consumable food source. Spirulina controls blood sugar levels, improves the immune system, reduces cholesterol and helps the body to absorb minerals.

Chlorella - Chlorella is a fresh water algae and contains a complete protein profile being more than 58% protein based.

Fruit Superfoods

Fruit superfoods are high in anti-oxidants and contain many phytochemicals, minerals and vitamins not available in vegetables. It is best to consume fruit as fresh & ripe as possible. But many of the fruit superfoods are not native to the United States, are shipped long distances and therefore are often in dehydrated or frozen form.

Goji Berries - Goji berries are distinctively flavored red berries containing more vitamin C than any other fruit. They host high levels of antioxidants making them an ideal natural whole food for reversing aging and protecting against disease. They contain 11 essential and 22 trace minerals, 18 amino acids, 6 essential vitamins, 5 essential fatty acids and numerous other phyto-chemicals and healthy nutrients.

Raw Cacao – Note that I lead with the word RAW. So, when you hear "chocolate is good for you" don't run to your local grocery store to buy a chocolate candy bar. Nearly all processed chocolates have been super-heated and contain unhealthy sugars and other chemical additives. Unfortunately, this chocolate no longer has the health benefits of Raw cacao and is actually downright dangerous for you.

The healthy "chocolate" is organic raw cacao. The cacao can be in a powder, nib or whole bean form. But above all other factors make sure your chocolate has not be over heated.

Raw cacao contains possibly the world's most concentrated source of fruit based antioxidants having a (ORAC) score of 95,500. Cacao is also high in magnesium, iron and essential fatty acids.

Acai – Acai contains powerful antioxidant properties primarily due to high levels of anthocyanins. The ORAC rating of acai is 1,027. Make sure to look for the freeze dried acai fruit in which the nutrients are kept intact. When buying acai juice, purchase a brand that has not pasteurized or heated the Acai in any way.

Pomegranate – Pomegranates contain antioxidants like polyphenols, tannins, and anthocyanins which are effective in removing free radicals. Research indicates that nutrients within pomegranates help prevent hardening of the arteries by reducing blood vessel damage.

Coconut Water - Young coconut water is one of the highest sources of electrolytes in nature. Electrolytes are ionized salts in our cells that transport energy throughout the body. Coconut water is a much better alternative to commercial sports drinks laden with artificial sugars and colors. The molecular structure of coconut water is identical to human blood plasma meaning it is immediately recognized by the body and put to good use. Drinking the water from a young coconut is like giving your body an instant blood transfusion. In-fact this was common practice during World War II in the Pacific where both sides in the conflict regularly used coconut water, siphoned directly from the coconut, to give emergency transfusions to wounded soldiers.

Noni - Noni contains a multitude of vitamins, minerals, enzymes and phytonutrients. It has anti-bacterial, anti-tumor activity, & anti-inflammatory properties. It is effective as a pain reliever, generates cell repair and strengthens the immune system. Noni is beneficial for digestive disorders, skin disorders, pain relief, headaches, infections and more. Avoid pasteurized products.

Bee Superfoods

Royal Jelly - Queen Bees feed exclusively on royal jelly. The beautiful queen bee lives for up to approximately six years. Worker bees, which eat only honey and pollen, live for only approximately six weeks! We should take a note from nature on this one.

Royal jelly is a natural substance from the bee hive that is composed of trace amounts of many life-giving nutrients and biologically active compounds including some of the following:
• B Complex Vitamin
• Amino Acids
• Minerals: Calcium, Magnesium, Potassium, and Zinc
• Peptides
• Monosaccharides and Disaccharides
• Nucleic Acids
• And much more

41

Bee Pollen – Bee pollen contains over 5,000 enzymes and co-enzymes which exceeds levels naturally present in other foods!

Bee pollen is the most complete food found in nature and has five to seven times more protein than beef.

Bee pollen is a concentrated source of the B vitamin complex, along with vitamins A, C, D, E, selenium, lecithin. Powerful phytochemicals makes bee pollen a potent source of antioxidants. It is also great for fighting allergies but typically only if you purchase local bee pollen.

Propolis - Propolis is the substance collected from various plants by bees. Propolis is scattered throughout the hive walls and coats every opening to form a perfect natural bacteria and virus barrier. It is primarily used as an antibiotic and believed to stimulate phagocytosis, the means by which white blood cells destroy bacteria. Propolis also works against viruses, something that antibiotics cannot do.

Seaweed Superfoods

Seaweeds absorb nutrients direct from the ocean and are the most nutritionally dense plants on the planet. Ounce for ounce they are higher in vitamins and minerals than any other food. Ocean vegetables also contain more protein than all other vegetable sources. Additionally, the structure of seaweed mimics human blood plasma perhaps making this their greatest benefit which is regulating and purifying our blood system. Seaweed available for human consumption include:

Nori – Kelp – Dulse – Arame – Wakame - Kombu

There may be more superfoods out there but these will change your life if you use them in one way or another on a daily basis.

Chapter 7

Variety Is The Spice Of Life

So one last point before we get to the recipes. We have all heard the old saying that "variety is the spice of life". When it comes to your food, I endorse this old saying.

There are many reasons that Americans are nutrient deficient. Eating mostly processed foods is the main reason. Items such as overcooking our foods, picking foods before they are fully matured, nutrient-depleted farmlands, excessive stress hormones that deplete nutrients and several more simple items are all contributing factors to declining health and nutrient deficiency issues.

But there is another reason, and I would dare say this may be one of the top reasons, that Americans are nutrient deficient:

Lack of Variety.

Have you ever wondered why even vegetarians and vegans get sick? Well one of the reasons they do get sick is because of a lack of variety. Most people, even vegetarians, eat primarily the same foods over and over. This reduction in variety of foods ultimately leads to a reduction of nutrient variety.

This imbalance or deficiency can be corrected very easily by continuously switching food sources and adding new items to your tables.

Unfortunately we eat the same foods month after month and year after year. In the modern world food is available year round through grocery stores and large international shipping companies and of course farms that are all over the planet. Before these massive companies existed, we were all forced to eat only those items that were in season or were stored after being harvested. So when the next season came around an entire new food group was made available and thus the body was flooded with different life giving nutrients.

So, instead of buying the same 38 foods when you go to your local stores simply pick up something new and different. Purchase seasonal foods harvested at peak ripeness. You never know what kind of fun and excitement will come your way when you step out of your old routines!

You can also grow some of your own produce. The most important reminder I can provide is to constantly add one if not more superfoods to your daily meals.

Part 4

The Culinary Delight Of High Speed Blending

Chapter 8

High Speed Recipes

Many of the recipes in *Living On High Speed* are original creations from my personal test kitchen and demonstration seminars. A few were given to me by some of my amazing Vita-Mix demonstration peers. Some of the following recipes were adapted from other high speed enthusiasts such as David Wolfe, Markus Rothkranz and Penni Shelton.

Living On High Speed is not a complete raw food reference guide. The recipes in this wellness guide are for high speed blenders. In the near future I will create a second raw/vegan cooking guide that will include many amazing raw and vegan recipes that can be made without a high speed blender.

Also, I have created the following chart as a starting recipe guide to help you begin your "Living On High Speed journey"! This chart contains the highest nutrient dense foods not including the superfoods that were discussed earlier. The foods on this chart are the highest rated foods created by Dr. Joel Fuhrman who created the "Aggregate Nutrient Density Index" (ANDI).

An ANDI score shows the nutrient density of a food on a scale from 1 to 1000. ANDI scores are calculated by evaluating a range of micronutrients including vitamins, minerals, phytochemicals and antioxidant capacities. The higher the concentration of these elements in a food per calorie the higher the score. Kale is a dark leafy green which has an ANDI score of 1000 while a soda has a score of 1.

Using The Quick Reference Chart - Chose 1 item from the Greens column and 1 or 2 items from the Fruit column and 1 item from the Liquid column and feel free to add optional items like Protein and Superfoods to create a complete nutritious and delicious meal. Within 45 to 70 seconds you will have the most nutrient dense smoothie / juice around.

			Optional	Optional
Greens	Fruit	Liquid	Protein	Super Foods
½ Cup Mustard Greens	1 Cup Strawberries	Young Coconut Water	Spirulina	Any from Chapter 6
1 Cup Watercress	1 Cup Pomegranate Juice	Fresh Vegetable Juice	Chlorella	Any from Chapter 6
1 Cup Kale	2 Plums	Fresh Celery Juice	Bee Pollen	Any from Chapter 6
½ Cup Turnip Greens	1 Cup Raspberries	Fresh Fruit Juice	Hemp Seeds	Any from Chapter 6
Collard Greens	1 Cup Blueberries	Pure Alkaline Water	Chia Seeds	Any from Chapter 6
2 Cup Spinach	½ Grapefruit	Pure Ice	Protein Powders	Any from Chapter 6
2 Cup Bok Choy	1 Orange		Pea, soy, whey	Any from Chapter 6
1 Cup Brussel Sprouts	1 Cup Cantaloupe			
	1 Kiwi			
	1 Cup Watermelon			
	½ Apple			
	1 Peach			

Add a "Daily Basic" Nutrient To Create A Perfect Meal!

Less Liquid To Thicken, More Liquid To Thin

To alkalize add: pinch sea salt, 1/8 tsp baking soda & 8 drops trace minerals

TIP - Avoid sugar of all types (including fruit) while dealing with issues such as bacteria overgrowth, candida, yeast problems, cancer and other sugar feeding diseases.

Now before getting to the recipes let's discuss just a few key points about juicing and making smoothies in your HSB.

Juicing In Your High Speed Blender

Here is an important juicing rule. Vegetables and fruits are not composed of enough liquid to make a great juice when blended on high speed. In fact, if you blend these items in a high speed blender you will likely create a wonderful paste, puree or sauce. (Think: Applesauce)

The easy fix - add enough liquid for the desired juice consistency. The more liquid you use the thinner the juice, the less liquid the thicker the juice. To thin my drinks and create some awesome juices I use pure filtered water or coconut water. But you can also use juices, milk or milk substitutes such as almond, soy, rice or other healthy milks.

Using ice will keep your drink cool and "live" by keeping the temp well below 115 degrees thus preventing enzymes from being denatured. But this will add additional liquid thus thinning out your drink. Two ways to avoid further thinning:
1. Add less liquid if you add ice.
2. Use frozen fruits or vegetables instead of ice.

CONSISTENCY ESTIMATES:
• No Liquid - Extra Thick (Like a Paste/Puree)
• ½ Cup Liquid - Thick (Like a Spaghetti Sauce)
• 1 Cup Liquid & ½ Cup Ice (to cool) - Medium (Like a Protein Smoothie)
• 1 ½ Cups Liquid & 1 Cup Ice - Thin (Like a V-8 or Odwalla drink)
• 2 Cups Liquid & 2 Cups Ice - Extra Thin (Like juice from a juice extractor)

Also please allow enough time for your high speed blender to emulsify all materials. Less than one minute of spin on high speed will likely leave trace amounts of "pulpy" fiber in-tact to a small extent. Running the machine on high speed for 2 or more minutes will ensure all fiber is small enough not to be noticed.

Yet another way to create a pulp free juice is by using a cheese cloth or nut-milk bag as a filter. High speed blenders are able to reduce skin, seeds, leaves and fiber down to a 95% bioavailability rate. This means that when blended for two to three minutes there will still be trace amounts of discernable fiber. These elements can be further removed by pouring the contents through a close knit cheese cloth or nut-milk bag, resulting in a fiber rich and nutrient dense drink that has zero "pulp". Thus with a HSB it is possible "to have your cake and eat it too!"

Smoothies:

Once upon a time there were no smoothies (at least not as we know them today). But in the late 1960's pioneer Steve Kuhnau, the founder of Smoothie King, began experimenting with mixing real fruits, super-food nutrients and different proteins in a blender at home with the intent to remedy low blood sugar levels and severe allergies that plagued him. He changed the world. Through the years the basics of a smoothie have remained the same by combining delicious fruits with many other nutrient dense elements like superfoods, vegetables, leafy greens, essential fatty acids and a myriad of protein sources.

In other words, smoothies have become not only a large part of American culture but also a mainstay in helping American's improve their health.

There are many variations and no wrong answers that can be applied when making your smoothies. You are only limited by your imagination. Now smoothies can be all fruit and nothing more than a delicious drink or they could be so nutrient dense that only diehards can drink them. But one thing is usually common regarding smoothies. They are naturally thick. Mostly because they are full of a large quantity of blended ice or other frozen produce, protein and other fibrous materials.

National smoothie outlets such as Smoothie King, Jamba Juice, Tropical Smoothie, Mawi Wowi and many others have become successful businesses and a popular smoothie source for many Americans. For some, these outlets are expensive. I have found cost to be as high as $5 to $9 per smoothie. Creating the same recipes at home typically ranges between $.75 and $4.00. Besides the cost, watch out for the ingredients. Some smoothie organizations use artificial syrups, flavors and additives to make those smoothies taste great. These additives are chemical-based which are of course not good for the body. Making smoothies at home can help you avoid these chemical compounds.

By the way, these professional smoothie organizations all use high speed blenders to get the job done. In my research I have found that 9 out of 10 smoothie companies use the Vita-Mix machine.

Now To Our Recipes Section

Smoothies & Juices

Notes

Use ice to chill, superfoods to thrive, use juice instead of water to enrich & thin your meal, add sweeteners to enjoy & add EFAs/protein of your choice to complete the meal, or leave as is!

Blend all recipes on high speed until smooth unless otherwise noted!

My Demo Recipes

Natural Pink Lemonade

- 2 to 3 Cups Red Grapes
- 2 to 3 Strawberries (with stems)
- 1 Wedge Fresh Lemon (the more lemon you use the tarter your lemonade will be)
- 1 to 1 ½ Cups Ice

Kale-Berry

- 1 Cup Strawberries
- 3 to 4 Kale Leaves with Stems
- 2 Cups Coconut Water

Carrot Tart

- 2 to 3 Carrots
- ½ Medium Apple
- ¼ to ½ Part of a Raw Beet
- 1 Small Piece of Fresh Ginger Root – To Taste
- 1 Small Piece of Lemon with Rind (optional and to taste)
- 1 Cup Water
- 2 to 3 Cups Ice

Mexican Vegetable Medley

- 1 Carrot
- 1 Tomato
- 1 Celery Stalk
- ¼ Onion
- ¼ to ½ Bell Pepper
- 1 Clove Garlic
- ¼ Cup Cabbage
- 1 TBSP/Cube Vegetable Based Organic Bullion
- 3 Stems Cilantro
- 2 Tbsp Mexican Spice
- 2 Cups Pure Water
- 1 Cup Ice

Shrek "Limey" Smoothie

Shrek Smoothie

- 1 to 2 Cups Green Grapes
- 1 Large Wedge of Pineapple with Core
- ½ Apple with Core
- ½ Banana
- 1 Large Handful of Fresh Spinach
- 1 Slice Lime
- Optional – Squeeze of Honey
- 2 Cups Ice

- 1 to 2 Cups Green Grapes
- 1 Large Wedge of Pineapple with Core
- ½ Apple with Core
- ½ Banana
- 1 Large Handful of Fresh Spinach
- Optional – Squeeze of Honey
- 2 Cups Ice

F8 Fruit Smoothie

- 1 to 2 Cups Green or Red Grapes
- 1 Large Wedge of Pineapple with Core
- ½ Apple with Core
- ½ to 1 Orange
- 1 Small Slice Kiwi (optional)
- 2 to 3 Strawberries
- ¼ to ½ Banana
- 1 to 2 Handful Blueberries
- 2 Cups Ice

Super Food Blues & Greens

- 1 to 2 Cups Green Grapes
- 1 Large Wedge of Pineapple with Core
- ½ Apple with Core
- ½ Orange
- 2 to 3 Strawberries
- ¼ Banana
- 1 to 2 handful blueberries
- 1 to 2 Tbsp of a Super Green Food (Spirulina, Chlorella, etc.)
- 2 Cups Ice

Refreshing Orange-Crème

- 1 ½ Cups Soy Milk
- 2 Tablespoons Pure Vanilla Extract
- 1 to 2 Large Oranges (Rind Removed)
- 2 Oz. Sugar in the Raw (or any sweetener of choice)
- 1 Cup Ice

Cabbagechino

- 1 ½ Cups Vanilla Flavored Soy Milk (or any milk of your choice)
- 1 Tablespoon Vanilla Extract
- 2 Oz. Sugar in the Raw (or any sweetener of choice)
- 2 Tablespoons Raw Cocoa
- 1 Teaspoon of Instant Or other ground coffee of your choice (add more if you like a strong coffee flavor)
- 1 Wedge Cabbage
- 1 to 2 Cups of Ice

Fresh Natural Soy Milk

- 2 to 3 Oz. Raw Soybeans
- 3 Cups Hot Water

Place raw dry soybeans in container before adding water. Blend on High Speed until powdered. Pour in hot water and blend on high speed for 6 to 7 minutes. Water will boil. Place hot liquid in refrigerator storage jar and refrigerate overnight.
Add flavoring and sweeteners (i.e. vanilla, sugar/honey or other) as desired during the blending process.

Chocolate/Peanut Butter Milk Shake

- ¼ to ½ cup nut butter (add if not already in the machine because you made fresh peanut butter)
- ½ to 1 cup coconut milk or other milk Substitute
- 1 Tablespoon Vanilla Extract
- 2 Oz. Sugar in the Raw (or any sweetener you prefer)
- 2 Tablespoons Cocoa
- 1 Wedge Cabbage (Optional)
- 1 to 2 Cups of Ice

Living Greens Smoothies

Smooth Alkalinity

- 1 Avocado
- 6 Figs
- 2 Cups of Baby Spinach
- 1 Cucumber
- 1 oz. Barley Grass Juice
- 1 ½ Cup Coconut Water

Dandelion Dream

- 2 Cups Dandelion Greens
- 1 Cup Pineapple
- 1 Banana
- ½ Apple
- 2 Cups Water

Dandy Anana

- 2 Cups Dandelion Greens
- 4 Bananas
- 1 Lime
- 2 cups water

Smooth Citrus Flax

- 4 Tbsp flax seeds
- 2 Oranges
- ½ Cup Pineapple
- 1 Banana
- 1 Cups Spinach
- ½ Cup Coconut Water

Jolly Green Giant

- 3 Cups Green Grapes
- ½ Cucumber
- ½ Cup Peas
- 1 Stalk Celery
- ½ Cup Broccoli
- ½ Avocado
- 1 oz. Wheat Grass Juice
- 1 Tbsp Raw Honey
- 1 Cup Coconut Water

Hairy Greens

- 2 Cups Spinach
- 1 Kiwi / skin
- 1 Cup Pineapple / Skin
- 1 Banana
- 2 Cups Water

Grassy Grapes

- 1 Cup Wheatgrass
- 2 Banana
- 1 Cup Green Grapes
- 2 Cups Water

Green Oranges

- 2 Small Oranges
- 1 Stalk Celery
- 7 Leaves Romaine
- 3-4 Kale Leaves
- 2 Banana
- 1 Pear
- 2 Cups Water

Peachy Greens

- 1 Bunch Spinach or Kale
- 2 Peaches or Nectarines
- 2 Cups Water

Fresh Roman

- 8 Leaves Romaine Lettuce
- 5 Cups Watermelon
- 1 Cup Water

Tangy Spinach

- 1 Cucumber
- 3 Celery Stalks
- 1 Handful Spinach
- 2 Tomatoes
- ½ Lemon
- 1 – 2 Cups Water

Green Roman

- 6 Leaves Romaine Lettuce
- 1 Cup Green Grapes
- 1 Medium Orange
- 1 Banana
- 2 Cups Water

Great Leaves

- 2 Aloe Vera Leaves
- 2 Oranges
- 1 Grapefruit
- 1 Lime
- 6 Kale Leaves
- 1 Cup Pineapple
- 3 Tbsp Any Green Superfood
- 1 cup water

Roman Honey

- 6 Leaves Romaine Lettuce
- ½ Honey Dew Melon
- 2 Cups Water

Mang-O-Lo

- 1 Cup Apple Juice
- 1 Banana
- 1 Mango
- 1 Aloe Leaf
- 5 Leaves of Kale
- 2 Cups Coconut Water

Cran-O-Lo

- 2 Aloe Vera Leaves
- 1-2 Cups Coconut Water
- Coconut Meat (optional)
- 1 Cup Cranberries
- 1 Bok Choy
- 2 Tbsp Herbs
- 2 Stalks Celery

Sweet Stinging Mango

- 4 Mangoes
- 1 Handful Stinging Nettles
- 4 Tbsp Raw Honey
- 2 Cups Water

Berry Roman

- 1 Cup Strawberries
- ½ Cup Blueberries
- 1 Banana
- 6 Romaine Lettuce Leaves
- 2 Cups Water

Cool Kiwi

- 2 Kiwis
- 1 Banana
- ½ Cucumber
- 2 Cups Water

Green Coconut

- 2 Cups Pineapple
- 1 Banana
- 1 Cup Coconut Meat
- 2 Cups Spinach
- 2 Tbsp Agave
- 2 Tbsp Coconut Butter
- 2 Cups Coconut Water
- 1 Tsp Spirulina
- 1 Tsp Vanilla Extract

Minty Pale

- 4 Pears
- 4 Leaves Kale
- 6 Mint Leaves
- 2 Cups Water

Smooth Spinach

- 3 Banana
- 2 Handful Spinach
- 2 Cups Water

Blue Green Aloe

- 3 Lettuce leaves
- ¼ Cup Sunflower Sprouts
- 1 Cup Spinach
- 1 Aloe Vera Leaf
- 6-7 Strawberries
- 1 Handful Blueberries
- 1 Cup of Coconut Water

Sweet Speer

- 2 Cups Pineapple
- 1 Cup Mango
- 1 Tsp. Vanilla Extract
- ¼ Cup Honey or Other Sweetener
- 2 Tsp Spirulina
- 1 Tbsp coconut butter
- 1 Young Coconut, Water & Meat
- 1 cup crushed ice

Cell-loe

- 1 Leaf Aloe Vera
- 2 Stalks Celery
- 2 Cups Kale
- ½ Apple
- 2 Banana
- 1 Lime
- 2 Cups Water

Berry Oxidant

- 1 Cup Raspberries
- 1 Cup Blueberries
- 2 bananas
- 1 big handfuls of baby spinach
- 2 cups of water

Tango

- ¼ Head of Green Lettuce
- 2 Tangerine
- ½ Cup Mango
- 1 Pear
- 1 Tbsp Kelp
- 1 cup of water

Orangano

- 1 Banana
- 1 Cup Bok Choy
- 6 Stems Oregano
- ½ Cup Grapes
- 1 Orange
- 1 Cups Water

Hot Mangos

- 1 Banana
- 3 Kale Leaves

Dandy Mint

- 2 Cups Dandelion Greens
- 10 Strawberries

- 2 Cups Mango
- Pinch of cayenne
- 1 Cup Almond Milk

- 2 Banana
- 5 Mint Leaves
- 2 Cups Water

Brawberry Greens

- ½ Cup Strawberries and Blueberries
- 1 Cup Spinach
- 1 Cup Mixed Greens
- 1 Cup Coconut Water
- ½ Cup Ice
- 1 Tbsp Wheat Germ
- ¼ Cup Coconut Meat
- ½ Tsp Honey

Goji Smooth

- ½ Cup Gojiberries
- 1 Cup Strawberries
- 1 Banana
- 1/2 bunch Romaine
- 1 Tbsp Raw Honey
- 2 Cups Water

Tai Blue Greens

- 1 Small Nectarines
- 1 Pears
- 1 Bananas
- 2 Cups of Greens
- 1 Tsb Blue Green Algae
- 1 Cup Coconut Water

Cucumber Chard

- 1 Cup Spinach
- 2 Stalks Celery
- 1 Cucumber
- 2-4 Chard Leaves
- 1 Banana
- 1 Peach
- ½ Cup Coconut Milk

Baby Broc

- 2 Broccoli Florettes
- ½ Kale Leaf
- 1 Celery Stalk
- 2 Baby Carrots
- ½ Apple
- 1 Cup water

Sweet Greens

- ½ Cup Pineapple Chunks
- ½ Mango
- 1 Banana
- 1 Carrot
- 1 Peach
- 2 Kale Leaves
- 2 Stalks Bok Choy
- 1 Broccoli Flouret

- 1 Stalk Celery
- 4 Dates
- 1 Tbsp Dulse
- 2 Cups Water

Pearly Green

- 1 Cup water
- Banana
- 2 Cups Grapes
- 1 Pear
- 2 Cups Spinach

Green Chocolate

- Dandelion Greens
- Mango
- 2 Bananas
- 8 Romaine Leaves
- 3 Tbsp Raw Cacao Powder
- 3 Tbsp Raw Honey
- 2 Cups Water

Bok Choy Joy

- 1 Bunch Bok Choy
- 1 Banana
- 1 Pear
- 6 Strawberries
- 1 Celery
- 1 Tbsp Flaxseed Oil
- 1 Cup Water

Orange Mint Greens

- 1 Lemon
- 1 Bunch Mint
- 1 Bunch Greens of Choice
- 2 Cups Orange Juice

Goji Mint

- 1 Banana
- ½ Cup Spinach
- ½ Bunch Mint
- 1 Tbsp Maca
- 3 Tbsp Chia Seeds
- 3 Tbsp Goji Berries
- 3 Dates
- 1 Cup Water

Raspberry Flax

- 1 Banana
- ½ Cup Raspberries
- 1 Pear
- 1 Cup Spinach
- 1 Tbsp Flax Seed
- 1 Cup Water

Sweet Rabbit Food

- ½ Apple
- ½ Peach
- 1 Nectarine
- 1 Carrot

Sweet Greens 2

- 3 Cups Mixed Greens
- 1 Celery Stalk
- 1 Cup Pineapple Juice
- 1 Banana

- ¼ Avocado
- 1 Lemon
- Handful Parsley
- Wedge Romaine Lettuce
- 1 cup water

- 1 Cup Water

Green Papa

- 1 Cup Baby Spinach
- 1 Bunch Parsley
- 2 Kale Leaves
- 1 Banana
- ½ Cup Pineapple
- 1 Cup Papaya
- ½ Mango
- 1 Tbsp Flax Seed
- 2 Cups Water

Strawberry Mint

- 1 Cup Spinach
- 4 Romaine Leaves
- 8 Mint Leaves
- 2 Cup Strawberries
- 1 Cup Water

Dull Bluberry

- 1 Cup Blueberries
- 1 Cup Spinach
- 1 Whole Carrot
- 1 Cup Water
- 1 Tbsp Dulse
- 1 Tbsp Coconut Meat
- 1/2 tsp Honey

Fat Orange

- 1 Orange
- 1 Cup Strawberries
- 1 Cup Carrot Greens
- 1 Tbsp Wheat germ
- 1 tsp Honey
- 1 Tbsp chia, hemp & Flax seeds
- 2 Cups Water

Mint Chocolate Kale

- 6 Kale Leaves
- 10 Mint Leaves
- 3 Bananas
- 2 Tbsp Carob Powder
- 3 Tbsp Raw Cacoa
- 2 Cups Water

Bok Choy Banana

- 3 Bananas
- ½ Bunch Dill
- 2 Celery Stalks
- 1 Cup Bok Choy
- 2 Cups Water

Sprouted Fat

Dark Blue Persimmon

- ½ Cup Spinach
- ½ Cup Alfalfa Sprouts
- 1 Tbsp Sprouted Chia Seeds
- 1 Tbsp Hemp Seeds
- 1 Cup Pineapple
- 1 Banana
- 1 Cup Water

- 2 Persimmons
- 1 Cup Spinach
- ½ Cup Dill
- 1 Tbsp Chlorella
- 2 cups of water

Super Hot

- 1 Celery Stick
- ½ Cucumber
- ¼ Ginger
- 3 Garlic Cloves
- 4 Sprigs Parsley
- 5 Mint Leaves
- 2 Tbsp Comfrey
- ½ Cup Dandelion Greens
- ¼ Cup Mushroom
- Pinch Coriander
- Barley Seed Sprouts
- 1 Tsp Tummeric
- 2 Cups Water

Chia Greens

- Hand Size Wedge Lettuce
- 1 Apple
- 1 Banana
- 1 Cup Dandelion Greens
- 1 Celery Stick
- 4 Tbsp Chia Seeds

Malp

- 1 Cup Mallow
- 1 Tbsp Algae
- ½ Cup Stinging Nettles
- 2 Pears
- 2 Banana
- 2 Cups Water

Beginners Delight

- ½ Cup Kale
- ½ Cup Spinach
- 1 Cup Green Grapes
- 1 Mango
- 1 Apple
- 1 banana
- ¼ Lime
- 2 Cups water

Minty Red Raspberries

- 3 Bananas
- 2 Mangoes
- 1 Cups Raspberries

Lemon Ginger Pears

- 1 cup spinach
- 1/2 inch ginger
- 1 lemon

- 1 Cup Red Grapes
- 5 Kale Leaves
- 5 Mint Leaves
- 1 Cup Water

- 1 cucumber
- 2 celery
- 2 pears
- 1 cup water

Parsed Grapes

- 3 Cups Grapes
- 1 Handful Parsley
- 1 Cup Water

Sweet & Sour

- 5 Kale Leaves
- 2 Lemons
- 1" Ginger
- 4 Tbsp Raw Honey
- 3 Tbsp Coconut Oil
- 1 Cup Coconut Water

Orange Red Greens

- 1 Cup Dandelion Greens
- ½ Cup Parsley
- ½ Cup Spinach
- 1 Banana
- 1 Orange
- 1 Cup Raspberries
- 1 Cup Water

Dragon Spinach

- 2 Bananas
- 1 Dragon Fruit
- 2 Cups Spinach
- 2 Cups of Water.

Sweet Sprouts

- 1 Cup Sprouted Wheat Seeds
- 1 ½ Cup Water
- 6 Dates

Not Green But Oh So Good!

Notes

Use ice to chill, superfoods to thrive, use juice instead of water to enrich & thin your meal, add sweeteners to enjoy & add EFAs/protein of your choice to complete the meal, or leave as is!

Blend all recipes on high speed until smooth unless otherwise noted!

Red White & Blue

- 6 Red Lettuce Leaves
- 3 apricots
- 1 banana
- ¼ cup blueberry
- 2 Tbsp Vanilla Powder
- 2 cups water

Chocolate Coco Milk

- 12 Cacao Beans
- 1 Coconut Meat & Juice
- 7 Cashews
- 1 big tablespoon coconut oil
- 3 Tbsp Raw Honey
- ½ Tsp Cinnamon
- Pinch Sea Salt
- Extra Coco Water as Needed

Smooth Chew

- 1 Avocado
- 4 Red Lettuce Leaves
- 3 Sprigs Parsley
- ½ Tsp Sea Salt
- ¼ Cup Cashews
- 1 Cup Coconut Water

Red Sweet Heat

- ½ Cup Goji Berries
- 2 Cups Pineapple
- ½ Cup Coconut Meat
- 2 Cups Red Grapes
- 2 Pinches Cayenne
- 1 Pinch Sea Salt

Pineapple Coconut

- 3 Cups Pineapple
- 1 Cup Coconut Meat
- 2 Tbsp Raw Honey
- 4 Tbsp Coconut Butter
- 2 Tbsp Vanilla Powder
- 2 Cups Coconut Water

Vanilla Banana

- 4 Bananas
- 4 Tbsp Vanilla Extract
- 2 Tbsp Raw Honey
- 2 Cups Rice Milk

Buzzn Chocolate Cherry

- 2 Cups Cherries
- 2 Cups Bananas

Cacoa Banana Cashew

- 4 Bananas
- 6 Tbsp Raw Cacao
- ¼ Cup Cashews
- 1 Tsp Cinnamon
- 2 Cups Coconut Milk
- ¼ Cup Raw Honey

Banana Berry

- 5 Cups Strawberries
- 2 Cups Bananas
- 1 Cup Soy Milk

Minty Cacao Smooth

- 1 Banana
- ½ Cup Coconut

- 8 Tbsp Raw Cacoa Powder
- 1 Tsp Bee Pollen
- 1 Cup Coconut Water
- 1 Tbsp Raw Honey
- 1 Tsp Vanilla Powder

- ¼ Cup Agave
- 2 Tbsp Vanilla Extract
- ¼ Cup Raw Cacao Powder
- 2 Cups Cashew Milk
- 10 Mint Leaves

Great Gojis

- 1 Grapefruit
- 2 Blood Oranges
- ¼ Cup Goji Berries
- 4 Strawberries
- 1 Tbsp Flax Seeds
- 1 Tbsp Chia Seeds

Nutty For Brazil

- 1 Cup Brazil Nuts
- 8 Dates
- 1 Tbsp Vanilla Extract
- 1 Cup Coconut Milk
- 1 Tbsp Kelp

Grape Pawpaw

- 1 Pawpaw
- 2 Cups Grape Fruit Juice
- 4 Mint Leaves

Vanilla Chocolate Nutmeg

- ¼ Cup Raw Cacao
- ½ Cup Raw Honey
- 1 Tbsp Vanilla Extract
- ½ Tbsp Nutmeg
- 2 Cup Almond Milk

Green Grapefruits

- 2 Bananas
- 1 Apple
- 2 Grapefruit
- 1 Tbsp Spirulina
- 4 Tbsp Hemp Seeds
- 2 Tbsp Chia Seeds
- 2 Tbsp Maca
- 1 Cup Grapfruit Juice

Watermelon Kiwi Cooler

- 2 Cups Watermelon
- 2 Kiwi
- 3 Strawberries
- 1 Cup Grapes
- ¼ Lime

Antioxidant Blues

- 1 Cup Blueberries
- 1 Cup Acai Juice
- 1 Cup Acai Berries
- 1 Banana

Fresh Fruit Smoothie

- 1 Cups Grapes
- 3 Strawberries
- ¼ Cup Blueberries
- 1 Piece Watermelon

- 2 Tbsp Honey
- ½ Cup Almond Milk

- 1 Cantaloupe Slice
- 1 Cup Pineapple
- 1 Banana
- 1 Apple
- 1 Cup Ice

Delicious Hot Cacao

- 1 Tbsp Raw Cacao Powder
- 1 Tbsp Maca Powder
- 2 Tbsp Raw Honey
- ½ Inch Ginger
- 1 Tsp Cinnamon
- 1 Cup Soy Milk

Limey Pineaplle

- 1 Cup Pineapple
- ½ Lime
- 1 Cup Apple Juice

Tangy Tomato

- 4 Large Tomatoes
- 1 Lemon
- 2 Celery Stalks
- 1 Tsp Braggs Aminos
- ¼ Tsp Cayenne Pepper
- ½ Tsp Sea Salt
- 1 Cup Water

Papa's Royal Straw

- 2 Cups Strawberries
- 1 Papaya Blended
- 1 Tsp Raw Honey
- ½ Tsp Bee Pollen
- ½ Tsp Royal Jelly
- 1 Cup Coconut Milk

Blueberry Lemonade

- 2 Cups Red Grapes
- 1/3 Lemon
- ½ Cup Blueberries
- 1 Cup Ice

Smooth Sesame Milk

- 1 Cup Sesame Seeds
- 1 Banana
- 3 Dates
- 1 Tbsp Vanilla Extract
- 2 Cups Water

Limey

- 2 Kiwis
- 1 Pear
- ½ Lime / Skin
- 2 Tbsp Raw Honey
- 1/4 cup water
- 1 cup ice

Royal Hemp

- 12 Cashews
- 2 Banana
- 2 Tbsp Hemp Seed
- 1 Tsp of Bee Pollen
- 1 Tbsp Honey
- ½ Tsp Royal Jelly

- 1 Tbsp Vanilla
- 2 Cups of fresh Coconut water

Canta-Berry

- 2 Cups Cantaloupe
- 1 Cups Strawberries
- 2 Cups Soy or Almond Milk

Pink Coconut Water

- ½ Medium Raw Beet
- 6 Dates
- 2 Tsp Vanilla
- 12 Strawberries
- 2 Tbsp Hemp Seeds
- 2 Tbsp Kefir
- 1 Cups Coconut Water

Tomato Mint

- 1 Bunch Parsley
- 5 Mint Leaves
- 1 Slice Onion
- ½ Lemon
- 2 Tomato
- 2 cups water

Blue Pomegranate

- 1 Large Pomegranate, seeded
- 1 Banana
- ½ Cup Blueberries
- 3 Tbsp Raw Honey
- 1 cup Soy or Almond Milk

Butternut Honey

- 1 Cup Butternut Squash
- 1 Tbsp Vanilla Extract
- 1/8 Tsp Cinnamon
- 1/8 Tsp Nutmeg,
- 1/8 Tsp Ginger
- 4 Tbsp Raw Honey
- 1 Cup Coconut Milk

Almond Apple Smooth

- 1 Apple
- 1 Pear
- 2 Bananas
- ½ Persimmon
- ½ Tsp Cinnamon
- ¼ Tsp Nutmeg
- 1 Cup Almond Milk

Roman Pineapple

- 1 Cup Pineapple
- 1 Pear
- 5 Leaves of Romaine Lettuce

Salsa Smoothie

- ½ Avocado
- 2 Tomatoes
- 1 Tsp Mexican Seasoning

- 1 Cup Coconut Water

- ½ Tsp Salt
- ½ Red Onion
- 4 Sprigs Cilantro
- 1 Orange Bell Pepper
- 1/8 Lime
- 2 Garlic Cloves
- 2 Tbsp Apple Cider Vinegar
- 2 Cups Water

Pink Cilantro

- 1 Pink Grapefruit
- ½ Cucumber
- 6 Sprigs Cilantro
- ½ Lime
- Vanilla Extract
- ½ Cup Water

Tomato Basil Smooth

- 4 Tomatoes
- 1 Red Bell Pepper
- 8 Basil Leaves
- ½ an Avocado
- 1/8 Tsp Salt
- 1 Cup Water

Tropical Coconut

- 2 Bananas
- ½ Mango
- 1 Papaya Solo
- 1 Cup Pineapple
- 1 Cup Coconut Water

Chocolate Seeds

- 1 Banana
- 1 Tbsp Hemp Seeds
- 3 Tbsp Cacao
- 1 Tbsp Maca
- 1 Tbsp Sesame Seeds
- 1 Tbsp Flax Seeds
- 2 Tbsp Raw Honey
- 1 Cup Coconut Water

Coco Carrot Tops

- 8 Carrot Top Greens
- ½ Avocado
- 1 Banana
- 4 Tbsp Coconut Oil
- 1 Cup Coconut Water

Maca / Carob Smooth Chew

- 3 Bananas
- 8 Cashews
- 1 Tsp Carob Powder
- 1 Tbsp Maca Powder
- 2 Tbsp Raw Honey
- 1 Cup Rice Milk

Orange / Pineapple Smooth

- 1 Cup Orange Juice
- 1 Cup Goat Yogurt

Papa Peach Smooth

- 1 Papaya Solo
- 1 Cup Peaches

- 1 Cup Pineapple

- 1/2 Cup Goat or Almond Milk
- 1 Tbsp Raw Honey

Coconut Colada

- ½ Cup Coconut Meat
- 1 Cup Pineapple
- 2 Tbsp Coconut Oil
- 1 Tsp Vanilla Extract
- 1 Tbsp Lime juice
- 4 Tbsp Raw Honey
- 1 Cup Coconut Water

Berry Chocolate

- 1 Cup Blueberries
- 2 Tbsp Raw Cacao
- 2 Tbsp Raw Honey
- 1 Cup Almond Milk

Pineapple GoGurt

- 1 Nectarine
- 1 Cup Goat Yogurt
- ½ Half Lemon / Skin
- 1 Cup Pineapple Juice
- 1/2 cup ice

More Than Sprouts

- 2 Bundles of Carrot Tops
- 2 Celery Stalks
- ½ Cup Alfalfa Sprouts
- 1 Aloe Vera Leaf
- 3 Bananas
- 1 Cup Grapes
- 2 Cups Water

Sweet Coriander

- 1 Bunch Coriander
- 1 Apple
- 1 Cup Grapes
- 1 Banana
- 1 Cup Water

Chocolate Cherry Shake

- 2 Cups Cherries
- 2 Bananas
- 4 Tbsp Raw Cacao Powder
- 1 Cup Coconut Water
- 1 Tbsp Raw Honey
- 1 Tsp Vanilla Extract
- 1 Cup Water

Peach Coco Smooth

- 1 Cup Peaches
- 1 Cup Goat yogurt
- 1 Cup Coconut Meat

Strawberry Banana Aloe Leaf

- 2 bananas
- 6-7 strawberries
- 1 Aloe Vera Leaf

- 1-2 Cup Coconut Milk
- Hand Sized Lettuce Wedge
- 1 cup water

Desserts

Notes:
Use ice, frozen fruit or frozen milk for ice creams & sorbets, to sweeten use healthy items such as raw sugar, Stevia, Zylitol, raw honey, juice or juice concentrates and use items like soaked chia seeds and pysillium to thicken your puddings.
Blend on high speed unless otherwise noted.

My Demo Dessert Recipes

"Bubble Gum" Sorbet

- ½ Cup 100% Juice
- ¼ Cup Raw Honey
- ½ - Banana
- 2 to 3 – Strawberries
- 1 Slice Pineapple
- 1 Serving – Red Cabbage (small handful)
- 3 Cups Ice

30 to 40 seconds on high speed

"Lime or Shrek" Sorbet

- ½ Cup 100% Juice
- ¼ Cup Raw Honey
- ¼ Banana
- 1 Slice Pineapple
- Handful Spinach
- 1 Wedge Lime
- 3 Cups Ice

30 to 40 seconds on high speed

Strawberry Ice Cream

- 1 Cup – Milk Substitute or Milk
- 2 to 3 ounces of Sugar in the Raw (or sweetener of choice)
- 1 tablespoon Vanilla Extract
- 1 Serving (fits in palm of your hand) – Red Cabbage & or 2 baby carrots

Vanilla Ice Cream

- 1 Cup – Milk Substitute or Milk
- 2 to 3 ounces of Sugar in the Raw (or sweetener of choice)
- 1 to 2 tablespoons Vanilla Extract
- 3 – 4 Cups Frozen Milk Substitute or Milk
- Or 2 to 3 Cups of Ice (using ice

- 4 Cups Frozen Strawberries

30 to 40 seconds on high speed

Banana Ice Cream

- Cup – Milk Substitute or Milk
- 2 to 3 ounces of Sugar in the Raw (or sweetener of choice)
- 1 to 2 tablespoons Vanilla Extract
- 2 to 3 Bananas
- 2 to 3 Cups Frozen Milk Substitute or Milk
- Or 2 to 3 Cups of Ice (using ice will make this slightly less creamy)

30 to 40 seconds on high speed

Chocolate Banana Ice Cream

- 1 Cup – Milk Substitute or Milk
- 2 to 3 Ounces of Sugar in the Raw (or sweetener of choice)
- 2 Tbsp Vanilla Extract
- 2 Banana's
- 2 to 3 Heaping Tablespoons of Raw Cocoa Or 6 oz Hershey's Unsweetened Chocolate Powder.
  • 2 to 3 Cups Frozen Milk Substitute or Milk
- Or 2 to 3 Cups of Ice (using ice will make this slightly less creamy)

will make this slightly less creamy)

30 to 40 seconds on high speed

Chocolate Ice Cream

- 1 Cup – Milk Substitute or Milk
- 2 to 3 ounces of Sugar in the Raw (or sweetener of choice)
- 1 to 2 tablespoons Vanilla Extract
- 2 to 3 Heaping Tablespoons of Raw Cacoa Or 6 oz. Nestle Quick Chocolate Drink Mix
- 3 – 4 Cups Frozen Milk Substitute or Milk
- Or 2 to 3 Cups of Ice (using ice will make this slightly less creamy)

30 to 40 seconds on high speed

Choco Banana Butter Cream

- 1 Cup – Milk Substitute or Milk
- 2 to 3 Ounces of Sugar in the Raw (or sweetener of choice)
- 2 Tbsp Vanilla Extract
- 2 Banana's
- 2 to 3 Heaping Tablespoons of Raw Cocoa Or 6 oz Hershey's Unsweetened Chocolate Powder
- 3 Tbsp Raw Peanut Butter
- 2 to 3 Cups Frozen Milk Substitute or Milk
- Or 2 to 3 Cups of Ice

Puddings

Green Mint Pudding

- 1 Cup Spinach
- 3 Banana
- 5 Mint Leaves
- 5 Dates
- 2 Tsp Psyllium Powder
- 1 Cup Coconut Water

Coconut Pudding

- 1 Coconut, Meat & Water
- 3 Tbsp Chia Seeds
- 1 Tsp Vanilla Extract
- 2 Tbsp Raw Honey
- Pinch Cinnamon
- Pinch Nutmeg
- ½ Cup Coconut Water

Green Vanilla Sauce

- 1 Cup Spinach
- 2 Banana
- ½ Apple
- 1 Vanilla Bean Or 2 Tbsp Extract
- ½ Small Lemon

Pers-Lemon Sauce

- 5 persimmons
- 1 Lemon
- 2 Cups Spinach
- 1 banana
- ½ teaspoon cinnamon
- ½ teaspoon nutmeg

Not As Healthy But Delicious

Blueberry Ice Cream

- ½ Cup Nut Cheese
- 2 Oz. Raw Sugar or Other Sweetener
- 1 Tbsp Vanilla Extract
- 3 Cups Frozen Blueberries
- 1 Cup Coconut Milk
- 1 Cup Frozen Coconut Milk

Choco/Carob Cream

- 2 Tbls Raw Cocoa
- 1 Tbsp Carob
- 2 Frozen Bananas
- ½ Cup Dates
- 1 Cup Almond Milk
- 3 Cups Frozen Almond Milk
- ½ Cup Any Nut Butter

Toffee Honey Delight

- 1 Frozen Toffee Bar
- ½ Cup Soy Milk
- 2 Cups Healthy Vanilla Ice Cream
- 1 Tbsp Raw Honey

Vanilla Peanut Butter Cup

- 2 Cups Healthy Vanilla Ice Cream
- ½ Cup Soy Milk
- ½ Cup Chunky Peanut Butter
- 2 Tbsp Raw Honey

Mocha Coco Cream

- ½ Cup Strong Coffee or 3 Tbsp Fresh Ground Coffee
- ½ Cup Coconut Milk
- 3 Tbsp Raw Cacoa
- 2 Tbsp Vanilla Extract
- 4 Tbsp Raw Honey
- 3 Cups Frozen Coconut Milk

Soups

Notes:

Keeping your soups below 115 degrees will keep the enzymes live and intact. Use less liquid to thicken, use more liquid to thin your soup base, use slower speed to add texture and use high speed to heat. The longer you spin on high speed the hotter the soup will become.

Tortilla Soup

- 1 Carrot
- 1 Celery Stalk
- 2 Roma Tomato
- 1 Slice Onion
- 1 Small Piece Yellow Squash
- 1 Wedge Green Cabbage
- 1 to 3 Slices Bell Peppers
- 1 to 3 Cloves of Garlic
- 5 Sprigs Cilantro
- 1 Slice of Jalapeno (size to taste)
- 3 Tbsp Sea Salt
- 1 to 2 Tbsp Mexican Spice
- 3 Cups Hot Water

Add ½ to 1 Cup Corn/Black Beans (pre-cooked)to soup after hot. Spin on slow speed.

Coco Mint Soup

- 1 Red Bell Pepper
- ½ Avocado
- 1 Cup Coconut Water
- 1 Celery Stalk
- 1" Pieces Ginger Root
- 10 Mint Leaves
- 3 Tbsp Seasoning To Taste

- 1 Handful Tortilla Chips

Stinging Netty

- 1 Cup Stinging Nettles
- 2 Celery Stalks
- ½ Cup Parsley
- 4 Garlic Cloves
- ½ Lemon
- 1 Potato
- 1 Avacado
- 2 Tbsp Sea Salt
- 2 Cups Water

Sweet Creamy Ginger

- 2 Cups Spinach
- 1 pear
- 6 Dates
- 1 Avocado
- 1" Ginger
- Pinch Sea Salt
- 2 Cups Water

Spicy Cilantro

- 2 Cups Cilantro
- 1 Celery Stalk
- 4 Romaine Lettuce Leaves
- 4 Tomatoes
- 1 Avacado
- 1 Lemon
- ½ Jalapeno
- Pinch Sea Salt
- 2 Cups Water

Oregano Dill Weed

- 1 Cup Dandelion Greens
- 1 Cucumber
- 1 Avacado
- 4 Garlic Cloves
- ½ Cup Dill Weed
- ½ Cup Oregano
- 1 Lime
- Pinch Sea Salt
- 2 Cups Water

Arugula Tart

- 2 Cups Arugula
- 1 Celery Stalks
- 4 Tomatoes
- 1 Avacado
- ½ Cup Basil
- ¼ Parsley
- 1 Lemon
- ½ Jalapeno
- Pinch Sea Salt
- 2 Cups Water

Mustard Cilantro

- 2 Cups Mustard Greens
- ½ Cup Cilantro
- 2 Tomatoes
- 1 Lime
- 4 Tbsp Spicy Mustard
- 1 Avacado
- 2 Cups Water

Sun Dried Spinach

- 1 Cup Spinach
- ½ Cup Dill
- ½ lime
- 3 cloves garlic
- 1 Cup Sun Dried Tomatoes
- 1 Tbsp Sea Salt
- 2 Cups Water

Basic Savory Green Soup Recipe

- 4 Tomatoes
- 3 Celery Stalks
- ½ Avocado
- ½ Bunch Parsley
- 1 Cup Spinach
- 2 Cups Orange Juice

Jalapeno Tomatoes

- 6 Roma Tomatoes
- 2 Cups Arugula Leaves
- ½ Jalapeno Pepper
- 4 Garlic Cloves
- ½ Tsp Cumin
- Pinch of Salt
- 2 cups water

Smokey Black Bean

- ½ Red Onion
- 1 Chipotle Pepper
- ½ Red Pepper
- ½ Green Pepper
- ½ Jalapeno Pepper
- 4 Garlic Cloves
- 1 Tbsp Cumin
- 1 Tsp Sea Salt
- ½ Tsp Black Pepper
- 2 Cups Soaked/Sprouted Black Beans
- 3 Cups Vegetable Broth

Tomato Vegetable

- 5 Tomatoes
- 1 Cup Cabbage
- ¼ Squash
- ½ Small Onion
- ¼ Cup Basil
- 4 Garlic Cloves
- Pinch Salt
- 1 Cup Vegetable Broth

Canta - Lime

- 1 Cantaloupe
- 1 Cup Orange Juice
- 1 Lime
- 6 Mint Sprigs

Taste Best If Chilled

Creamy Turnip

- 1 CUP Goat Yogurt
- 2 Leeks
- 1 Cooked Potato
- 3 Turnips
- 3 Tbsp Earth Balance Butter
- 2 Cups Vegetable Broth
- Pinch of Sea Salt

Black Bean

- 1 Cup Soaked Raw Black Beans
- 1 Cup Soaked Raw Chickpeas
- ½ Onion
- 4 Garlic Cloves
- ½ Jalapeno
- 1 Tsp Cumin
- 1 Tsp Chili Powder
- 2 – 3 Cups Water or Vegetable Broth

Add the following on low speed after soup has reached desired temp
- ¼ Cup Soaked Black Bean
- ¼ Cup Soaked Chickpeas
- ½ Cup Bell Pepper Assorted Color
- ¼ Scallions

Carrot Ginger Smooth

- 3 Carrots
- ¼ Onion
- 4 Garlic Cloves
- 1" Ginger
- ½ Tsp Salt
- ¼ Tsp Pepper
- 2 Cups Vegetable Broth

Apple Butternut Squash

- 2 ½ Cups Butternut Squash
- ¼ Onion
- 1 Garlic Clove
- ¼ Lentils
- 1 Apple
- ¼ Tsp Thyme
- ¼ Tsp Salt
- 2 Cups Water or Vegetable Broth

Curried Carrot

- 6 Carrots
- ½ Onion
- ½ Cup Soy Milk

Sweet Potato

- 1 Sweet Potato
- 1 Tomato
- ½ Apple

- 2 Tsp Curry

- 1 Carrot
- ¼ Tsp Salt
- 2 Cups Water or Vegetable Broth

Cream Of Spinach

- 3 Cups Spinach
- ¼ Cup Onions
- 1 Tsp Cornstarch
- 4oz. Firm Tofu
- 1 Tsp Olive Oil
- 2 Cups Vegetable Broth

Pinto Bean Soup

- 1 Cup Soaked Pinto Beans
- ¼ Onion
- ¼ Tsp Salt
- 1/8 Tsp Pepper
- 1 Clove Garlic
- 2 Cups Water or Vegetable Broth

Tomato Tofu

- 2 Tomatoes
- ½ Onion
- 1 Cup Soy Milk
- 12oz. Firm Tofu
- 4 Basil Leaves
- ½ Tsp Salt
- ½ Tsp Pepper
- 1 Tbsp Olive Oil

Sweet Pea

- 1 Cup Peas
- ¼ Bell Pepper
- 1 Carrot
- ¼ Onion
- ¼ Tsp Salt
- 1/8 Tsp Pepper
- 1 Clove Garlic
- 2 Cups Water or Vegetable Broth

Appetizers, Dips, Spreads & More

Notes

Use sweeteners sparingly, avoid processed sugars and use natural sweeteners like honey, stevia, dates & etc.

Blend on high speed unless otherwise noted.

Mango Salsa

- 1 Tomatilla
- 2 Cloves Garlic
- Slice of Onion
- 1 Slice of Green, Red, Orange and Yellow Bell Pepper
- Fresh Cilantro to Taste (Leaves only)
- 2 1/8" Slices of Fresh Mango
- 1 Tbsp Apple Cider Vinegar
- Squeeze of Lime
- 2 Shakes of Mexican Spice (cumin based)

Blend garlic and tomatilla on high speed. Add remaining elements and blend on low speed for 30 seconds.

Demo Salsa

- 1 Tomatilla
- 2 Cloves Garlic
- Slice of Onion
- 1 Slice of Green, Red, Orange and Yellow Bell Pepper
- Fresh Cilantro to Taste (Leaves only)
- 1 Slice Jalapeno (size to taste)
- 1 Tbsp Apple Cider Vinegar
- Squeeze of Lime
- 2 Shakes of Mexican Spice (cumin based)

Blend garlic, jalapeno and tomatilla on high speed. Add remaining elements and blend on low speed for 30 seconds.

Medium To Hot Salsa

- 1 Tomatilla
- 2 Cloves Garlic
- Slice of Onion
- 1 Slice of Green, Red, Orange and Yellow Bell Pepper
- Fresh Cilantro to Taste (Leaves only)
- 1 to 2 Jalapenos
- 1 Tbsp Apple Cider Vinegar
- Squeeze of Lime
- 2 Shakes of Mexican Spice (cumin based)

Blend garlic, jalapeno and tomatilla on high speed. Add remaining elements and blend on low speed for 30 seconds.

Mexican Spread

- 1 Cup Goat Cheese
- 1 Cup Sour Cashew Cheese
- 1 Tsp Cayenne
- 1 Tbsp Cumin
- 1 Tsp Jalapeno
- 1 Tsp Oregano
- 1 Tsp Paprika
- 4 Sprigs Cilantro

Lime Green Apple Sauce

- 1 Handful Spinach
- 2 Apples
- ½ Lime
- 1 Banana

High speed for 30 seconds.

Raw Apple Sauce

- 2 Apples
- 2 Bananas

High speed for 30 seconds.

Guacamole

- 2 Avocados
- ½ Lemon
- 2 Tbsp Chopped Onions
- ½ Tomato Chopped
- ½ Tsp Salt
- 2 Tbsp Olive Oil

Low Speed 10 to 15 seconds.

Green Banana-Berry Sauce

- 2 Banana
- Handful of Strawberries
- Large Handful of Spinach
- Dab of Water

High speed for 30 seconds.

Hot Guacamole

- 1 Tomato
- ½ Onion
- 3 Avocados
- 2 Garlic Cloves
- ½ Tsp Cayenne or Other Hot Spice
- Pinch Salt
- 2 Tsp Lemon Juice

Low Speed 10 to 15 seconds.

Orange Marinade

- ½ Cup Orange Juice
- 4 Garlic Cloves
- 1 Lime
- ½ Tsp Cumin
- ¼ Cup Cilantro Leaves
- ½ Tsp Dried Oregano
- ½ Mango
- 3 Tbsp Raw Honey
- 1 Tsp Salt and Black Pepper

Blend on high speed until smooth.

Spinach Dip

- 1 Cup Goat Yogurt
- ½ Cup Mayonnaise (that you created)
- 1 Cup Spinach
- 1 Package Healthy Vegetable Dry Soup Mix

Blend on medium speed.

Basil Pesto Sauce

- 2 Cups Basil Leaves
- 2 Garlic Cloves
- ¼ Lemon
- ¾ Cup Olive Oil
- ½ Tsp Oregano
- ¼ Cup Parsley
- ½ Cup Cashew Cheese
- Pinch Salt and Pepper

Blend on high speed.

Tropical Fruit Dip

- ½ Cup Almond Milk
- 1 Cup Cashew Cheese
- ½ Gelled Chia Seeds
- 6 Tbsp Coconut Meat
- 3 Tbsp Raw Honey
- 1 Cup Pineapple

Sweet Cream Dip

- 1 Cup Cashew Cheese
- 3 Oz Turbinato Sugar
- 5 Tbsp Raw Honey
- 1 Tbsp Vanilla Extract

Hot and Spicy Marinade

- 1" Slice Jalapeno
- 5 Pepperoncini
- 3 Shallots
- 1 Tbsp Allspice
- 5 Cloves
- ½ Cup Apple Cider Vinegar
- 1 Lime
- 3 Oz. Turbinato Sugar
- 1 Tsp Black Pepper
- ½ Saflower or Coconut Oil

Raw Red Pepper Hummus

- 3 Tbsp Olive Oil
- ½ Lemon
- 6 Tsp Sesame Seeds
- 1 Cup Soaked Garbanzo Beans
- ¼ Red Bell Pepper
- 2 Garlic Cloves
- 1 1/8" Slice Onion
- 1 Tsp Cumin
- 1 Tsp Salt
- ½ Tbsp Parsley
- 1 Tbsp water

Maple Date Sauce

- 1 Cup Maple Syrup
- 2 Tbsp Vanilla Extract
- 10 Dates
- ¼ Lemon
- 3 Tbsp of Water
- Pinch of Salt

Cilantro Chili Sauce

- 2 Tbsp water
- ½ Cup Raw Honey
- 1 Jalapeno
- 1 Cup Cilantro Leaves

Cucumber Yogurt Spread

- 2 Cups Goat or Greek Style Yogurt
- 1 Cucumber
- 2 Tbsp Sea Salt
- 5 Garlic Cloves
- 2 Tbsp Apple Cider Vinegar
- 3 Tbsp Olive Oil
- 12 Fresh Mint Leaves
- 1 Tsp Black Pepper

Herbed Butter

- 1 Cup Earth Balance
- 9 Garlic Cloves
- 1 Cup Parsley
- ¼ Cup Thyme
- ¼ Cup Oregano
- ¼ Cup Rosemary
- ¼ Cup Chives
- 1 Tbsp Salt

Strawberry Butter

- 1 Cup Earth Balance Butter
- 1 Cup Strawberries
- 3 Tbsp Raw Honey

Blend on medium speed.

Honey Butter with Cinnamon

- 1 Cup Earth Balance Butter
- 3 Tbsp Honey
- 1 Tsp Cinnamon

Blend on medium speed.

Celery Seed Dressing

- 2/3 Cup Agave Nectar
- 5 Tbsp Apple Cider Vinegar
- 1 Tbsp Lemon Juice
- 1 Tsp Dry Mustard
- 4 Tsp Onion

Bean Spread

- 1 Cup Sprouted Cannellini Beans (any beans will do)
- ¼ Cup Parsley
- 2 Tbsp Fresh Lemon Juice
  1 Tbsp Olive Oil

- 1 Tsp Salt
- 1 Tsp. Celery Seed
- 1 Cup Olive Oil

- 3 Garlic Clove
- Pinch Salt a
- Pinch Pepper
- 2 Tbsp Olive Oil

A Word on Nut Butters and Nut Cheeses

Nut Butters	Nut Cheeses

Nut Butters

Raw nuts are healthier but roasted nuts blend into creamier nut butters. Delicious butters can also be made from seeds.

Some nuts contain the proper amount of oil to create smooth creamy nut butters while others require the addition of a little oil to the mixture. The oil will separate from the nut butter once you store it. You can skim the oil off the top or stir it back into your nut butter.

Try to use the same oil as the nut you are blending or use neutral flavored oils like safflower oil.

A healthier option (than adding oil) is to soak your nuts in water before blending. Simply remember that soaked nuts render a different texture than non-soaked nuts.

A note for seeds: sesame, hemp, sunflower and pumpkin seeds are also

Nut Cheeses

Nut cheeses are healthy nondairy cheese alternatives. Does this seem weird? Well don't knock it before you try a few options.

White nuts like cashews, pine, almonds, macadamia work best but all other nuts and even seeds work well. Use the below recipes and ideas as a basic guide.

It is best to soak nuts before mixing but not mandatory.

You can ferment or "sour" your cheese one of three ways.

1. Allowing nut butters to sit for 12 or more hours in a warm area before enjoying.
2. Adding probiotics to your nut butters and allowing the butter to sit for 12 hours before enjoying.
3. Adding lemon and salt and enjoying immediately.
4. Add any other spices to add

good choices. However, use caution with these types of seeds. Their oils tend to be volatile and will quickly become rancid. It only takes a few "bad seeds" to ruin of whole batch of seed butter.

flavor to your cheeses

Peanut Butter

- 3 Cups Raw Peanuts
- Optional 3 Tbsp Honey

Blend on high speed until smooth. About 90 seconds to 2 minutes. *Don't Over Process*

Macadamia Cheese

- 2 Cup raw Macadamia Nuts
- 1 to 1 ½ Cup Water
- After blending to a smooth texture, let sit for 12 hours, add probiotics or add seasoning or do all three to enrich the flavor

Almond Butter

- 3 Cups Raw Almonds

Blend on high speed until smooth.

Chick Cheese

- ½ Cup Sprouted Chick Peas
- ½ Cup Water
- ½ Lemon
- 1 Tbsp Chives
- 1 Tbsp Oregano

Blend on high speed until smooth.

Cashew Butter

- 3 Cups Raw Cashews
- 3 Tbsp Oil

Blend on high speed until smooth.

Almond Cheese

- 2 Cups Raw Almonds
- 1 ½ Cup Water or Coconut Water
- ½ tsp Salt
- Juice From One Lemon

Blend on high speed until smooth.

Honey Maple Nut Butter

- 1 Cups Earth Balance Butter
- ¼ Cup Raw Honey

Cashew Cheese

- 2 Cups Raw Cashews

- ¼ Cup Maple Syrup
- 2 Cups Nuts Of Choice
- ½ Tsp Nutmeg
- Pinch Cinnamon
-

Blend on high speed until smooth.

- 1 to 1 ½ Cup Water
- ½ Lemon
- 1 Tbsp Chives
- 1 Tbsp Oregano

Blend on high speed until smooth.

Dried "Parm" Cheese

- 1 Cup Chopped/Powdered Walnuts
- ½ Tbsp Dried Garlic
- 1 Tsp Seal Salt
- 1 Sun Dried Tomato, Powdered

Stir Together

Part 5

Your Body On High Speed

Chapter 9

High Speed Workouts

Although eating properly is the first and best step toward regaining your health and achieving optimal performance, it is not the last.

In-fact achieving a healthy balance both on the inside and outside has several facets, most of which will be covered in a later chapter. Knowing, understanding and implementing the philosophy of "moving your body" or "working out" is the second most important aspect of regaining your health. There are several perspectives on moving the body otherwise known as "working out" two of which I will highlight in this section: resistance training and cardio training. Later in the book I will also discuss several other aspects of moving your body.

Resistance Training:

The most well known resistance training is Weight Training. This includes using dumbbells, barbells, fluids, pressurized air, elastic devices, springs, and a host of other devices designed to provide external resistance to one's musculoskeletal system. There are also several special forms of resistance training which are known as light training. Running, swimming, plyometrics, dance, calisthenics are all special workout forms designed to strengthen the body.

With regards to getting in great shape, the idea to hit the gym usually pops into mind. This thought of joining a gym prevents millions of people from achieving a healthy body. Over the years I have heard hundreds of people tell me why they cannot make it to the gym. Have you ever heard any of the following excuses? "I can't afford it", "I don't want to look beefy", "I don't have time", "I have children"?

But there is good news! You don't have to join the gym to get in great shape. The term working out just means MOVE YOUR BODY or GET TO WORK, not, get to the gym! In some parts of the world people still move their bodies from sunrise to sunset. However, in more developed communities manual labor has been replaced by machines, robots and computers.

So what is a person to do? The answer is simple. Start using your body! In the great outdoors preferably! Find something you love like playing tennis, dancing or gardening and do it.

Here are just a few reasons why working out is the second most important element to improving your health.

- Helps to reduce the loss of muscle tissue as you get older. Did you know that on the average we lose 7% of lean muscle mass every 10 years?
- Helps to maintain a stable metabolism. For every one pound of muscle lost, your basal metabolic rate is lowered by fifty calories per day. This means that as you lose muscle you would have to automatically reduce how much you eat. This is impossible to maintain effectively and it is not healthy.
- Helps to maintain bone density.
- Helps to maintain flexibility.
- Helps to maintain a youthful appearance.
- Helps to maintain a correct posture.
- Helps to maintain circulation.
- Helps to maintain a healthy heart. And in doing so creates greater blood flow to the extremities allowing individuals to reduce their risk of cancer, heart disease and diabetes.

Now what happens if you cannot get outside or make it to your local gym or perhaps you cannot think of a physical activity that suits you? Don't worry about it because I can help! I have an alternative for you.

Visit www.livingonhighspeed.com for details. I have over 130 workout programs all of which can be used in the comfort of your home. 90 of these programs have resistance based training concepts. I probably have something to fit your particular need or desire.

Before we show you these workouts, let's discuss what "cardio" is and how it may help.

Cardio:

"Cardio" refers to cardiovascular, also known as aerobic exercise, is any physical exercise that improves one's cardiovascular or "oxygen" system resulting in a stronger heart, improved blood flow, improved lung capacity, more oxygen entered into the blood stream. Aerobic means "with oxygen" and refers to the use of oxygen in the body's metabolic or energy-generating process. Many types of exercise like swimming, dancing, running, biking, and plyometrics are aerobic, and by definition are performed at moderate levels of intensity for extended periods of time.

Cardio based exercises are the bane of existence for many, but yet an awesome endorphin high for others! Cardio exercises are both loved and hated worldwide.

But regardless of your love / hate relationship with cardio, there is no doubt that if applied properly, cardio is very good for your body and your mind!

Here's even better news. It was previously thought that cardio workouts needed to be long and tedious. But that is no longer the case. Modern training advice and scientific technology has shown us that there is a very large array of cardio exercises that require only 20 minutes to perform and can reduce fat stores by over 300%.

This style of training is called HIIT or High Intensity Interval Training. Think of it this way- run / swim / bike / dance / roller blade / aerobic workouts and etc. at a brisk rate (after a proper warm up of course) for about 60 seconds. Then sprint for about 30 to 60 seconds. Back off and repeat this sequence for as long as you can. No more than 20 minutes is normally needed. The above is not a 100% scientific definition, just a basic description.

Many programs I offer like Insanity, Turbo Jam and Turbo Fire are designed as HIIT training styles and will give you intense HIIT fat reductions. HIIT style training is more intense but the results are well worth the efforts!

Cardio Exercise:
- Burns fat.

- Elevates heart rate – i.e. builds a stronger heart.
- Tones muscles.
- Helps clean the Lymphatic system.
- Builds stamina.

Now let's take a closer look at what in-home workout programs I can offer to help you achieve your goals. I have grouped each program by type.

Weight Loss Programs

Program Name	Trainer	Workout Duration	Benefits	How It Works
Slim in 6®	Debbie Siebers	25–50 minutes	Full-body slimming and toning focused on abs, thighs, buns, and hips.	Combines cardio with light resistance moves to burn fat and reshape your body in 6 weeks.
Turbo Jam®	Chalene Johnson	20–45 minutes	Calorie burning and total-body sculpting focused on abs and thighs.	Kickboxing and body sculpting to the hottest tunes to burn more calories than almost any other exercise.
RevAbs™	Brett Hoebel	15–45 minutes	Fat-burning cardio, muscle-building and sculpting focused on abs and core.	Abcentrics™, Capoeira, cardio intervals, strength training, and ab/core work to get you six-pack abs in 90 days.
Brazil Butt Lift®	Leandro Carvalho	30–50 minutes	Reduce your hips, slim your thighs and lift your butt while you burn fat and melt away saddlebags.	Combines Brazilian dance, cardio, and signature sculpting moves with Leandro's proven TriAngle Training method that works your butt from multiple angles.
Power 90®	Tony Horton	35–45 minutes	Fat burning and total-body sculpting focused on abs, thighs, and upper body.	90-day boot camp featuring fast and effective circuit-training workouts to transform your body in as little as 35 minutes a day.
Rockin' Body®	Shaun T	15–45 minutes	Calorie-burning cardio and full-body sculpting moves.	Party off the pounds as you dance and sweat to the hottest hits of all time.
Hip Hop Abs®	Shaun T	25–45 minutes	Calorie-burning cardio and total-body sculpting focused on abs and core.	Fun hip hop dance moves set to hot music to burn fat and sculpt lean sexy abs.

Getting Started / Beginner Programs

Program Name	Trainer	Workout Duration	Benefits	How It Works
Turbo Jam®	Chalene Johnson	20–45 minutes	Calorie burning and total-body sculpting focused on abs and thighs.	Kickboxing and body sculpting to the hottest tunes to burn more calories than almost any other exercise.
Slim in 6®	Debbie Siebers	25–50 minutes	Full-body slimming and toning focused on abs, thighs, buns, and hips.	Combines cardio with light resistance moves to burn fat and reshape your body in 6 weeks.
Rockin' Body®	Shaun T	15–45 minutes	Calorie-burning cardio and full-body sculpting moves.	Party off the pounds as you dance and sweat to the hottest hits of all time.
Power 90®	Tony Horton	35–45 minutes	Fat burning and total-body sculpting focused on abs, thighs, and upper body.	90-day boot camp featuring fast and effective circuit-training workouts to transform your body in as little as 35 minutes a day.

Yoga Booty Ballet® Ab & Butt	Gillian Marloth & Teigh McDonough	35 minutes	Calorie burning and full-body sculpting focused on abs and booty.	Combines ab-sculpting yoga, booty-lifting ballet, and fat-melting cardio for total-body results while targeting your core and lower body.

Advanced Programs

Program Name	Trainer	Workout Duration	Benefits	How It Works
INSANITY®	Shaun T	30–60 minutes	Transform your body in 60 days with the most intense workout program ever put on DVD.	MAX Interval Training—you perform long bursts of maximum-intensity exercise with short periods of rest.
One on One with Tony Horton	Tony Horton	45–60 minutes	Effective home workouts for every part of your body.	Every month, Tony delivers his latest workout from his home to yours.
P90X® Plus	Tony Horton	20–45 minutes	The next level of advanced total-body training to get you ripped beyond belief.	Intense new cardio, muscle chiseling, and ab-/core-ripping moves to incorporate with P90X to ramp up your results.
Hip Hop Abs® Ultimate Results	Shaun T	30–45 minutes	Advanced cardio and body-sculpting moves targeting abs and core.	High-energy dance moves set to hip hop music for cardio, strength, and advanced ab sculpting.
ChaLEAN Extreme®	Chalene Johnson	30–45 minutes	Advanced circuit training program develops lean, sexy muscle to help you burn up to 60% of your body fat for overall body transformation.	The proven 3-phase circuit training technique is guaranteed to give you results every 30 days—the more muscle you build, the more fat your burn because Muscle Burns Fat®!
Turbo Jam® Fat Burning Elite	Chalene Johnson	30–50 minutes	Advanced kickboxing and body-sculpting moves focused on core, thighs, and upper body.	More intense targeted workouts to maximize your fat-burning and sculpting results.
Chalene Johnson's Get On the Ball!	Chalene Johnson	45–60 minutes	Advanced cardio and total-body sculpting focused on abs, core, and obliques.	Innovative moves with the Turbo Ball force your core muscles to work harder for fast, effective body transformation.
Slim Series® Express	Debbie Siebers	35 minutes or less	Advanced body slimming and toning focused on abs, thighs, butt, and hips.	Combines intense cardio with greater resistance to continue slimming and toning your body in under 35 minutes a day.
Yoga Booty Ballet® Master Series	Gillian Marloth and Teigh McDonough	20–35 minutes	Advanced sculpting workouts focused on abs, thighs, and booty.	Yoga and Pilates moves designed to target your abs and booty in special workouts for any time of day.
Power 90® Master Series	Tony Horton	50 minutes	Advanced total-body workouts focused on core, legs, hips, and glutes.	Targeted, innovative new cardio and sculpting moves to get you lean and ripped in less time.

Express (Time Saving) Programs

Program Name	Trainer	Workout Duration	Benefits	How It Works
10-Minute Trainer®	Tony Horton	10 minutes	Full-body workout in only 10 minutes a day.	Combines fat-burning cardio, total-body sculpting, and ab moves all at the same time for maximum efficiency!
Slim Series® Express	Debbie Siebers	35 minutes or less	Advanced body slimming and toning focused on abs, thighs, butt, and hips.	Combines intense cardio with greater resistance to continue slimming and toning your body in under 35 minutes a day.
Yoga Booty Ballet® Master Series	Gillian Marloth and Teigh McDonough	20–35 minutes	Advanced sculpting workouts focused on abs, thighs, and booty.	Yoga and Pilates moves designed to target your abs and booty in special workouts for any time of day.
Turbo Jam® LIVE!	Chalene Johnson	30 minutes	Calorie burning and targeted body toning focused on abs and booty.	Live classes with fun dance-party feel for slimming and sculpting and rockin' results.
Power Half Hour®	Tony Horton	30 minutes	Targeted body shaping focused on abs, arms, buns, and thighs.	Combines both cardio and targeted body sculpting for maximum results in just 30 minutes a day.
Great Body Guaranteed!™	Tony Horton and Debbie Siebers	under 10 minutes	Targeted body shaping focused on abs, arms, buns, and thighs.	Each move targets a specific zone to tighten and tone in under 10 minutes a day.

Specialty Programs

Program Name	Trainer	Workout Duration	Benefits	How It Works
Kathy Smith's Project: YOU! Type 2™	Kathy Smith	20–60 minutes	The first all-in-one, simple solution to help manage type 2 diabetes.	Helps prevent and control type 2 diabetes by providing an easy-to-follow, step-by-step nutrition plan and exercise program that works for all fitness levels!
Total Body Solution™	Debbie Siebers	15 minutes	Help relieve pain in your neck, shoulders, core, lower back, and knees.	These easy-to-follow drills will help relieve pain and prevent strain to get you back to your active lifestyle.

Get Real with Shaun T™	Shaun T	25–30 minutes	Cardio and strength training for kids ages 9 and up.	Have a blast as you alternate daily cardio and strength training workouts to manage weight and fitness.
Fit Kids® Club	Shaun T	25 minutes	Fun workouts for kids 7 and up to burn calories and get fit.	Light cardio and fun choreography to get kids of all shapes and sizes up and moving.
Tony & the Kids!	Tony Horton	30 minutes	Fun and simple moves for kids 5 and up to improve their coordination, balance, and flexibility.	Combines stretching, hopping, jumping, kicking, and twisting to help burn off kids' excess energy.
Tony & the Folks!	Tony Horton	30 minutes	Low-impact exercise for anyone age 55 and up.	A fun way to increase energy, reduce joint stiffness, and improve flexibility, strength, and balance.

Extreme Results Programs

Program Name	Trainer	Workout Duration	Benefits	How It Works
INSANITY®	Shaun T	30–60 minutes	Transform your body in 60 days with the most intense workout program ever put on DVD.	MAX Interval Training—you perform long bursts of maximum-intensity exercise with short periods of rest.
P90X®	Tony Horton	45–60 minutes	Advanced total-body training program focused on abs, legs, chest, back, and arms.	Twelve routines that keep introducing new moves and challenging your muscles to get you absolutely ripped in 90 days.
P90X® Plus	Tony Horton	20–45 minutes	The next level of advanced total-body training to get you ripped beyond belief.	Intense new cardio, muscle chiseling, and ab-/core-ripping moves to incorporate with P90X to ramp up your results.
One on One with Tony Horton	Tony Horton	45–60 minutes	Effective home workouts for every part of your body.	Every month, Tony delivers his latest workout from his home to yours.
RevAbs™	Brett Hoebel	15–45 minutes	Fat-burning cardio, muscle-building and sculpting focused on abs and core.	Abcentrics™, Capoeira, cardio intervals, strength training, and ab/core work to get you six-pack abs in 90 days.
ChaLEAN Extreme®	Chalene Johnson	30–45 minutes	Advanced circuit training program develops lean, sexy muscle to help you burn up to 60% of your body fat for overall body transformation.	The proven 3-phase circuit training technique is guaranteed to give you results every 30 days—the more muscle you build, the more fat your burn because Muscle Burns Fat®!

Chalene Johnson's Get On the Ball!	Chalene Johnson	45–60 minutes	Advanced cardio and total-body sculpting focused on abs, core, and obliques.	Innovative moves with the Turbo Ball force your core muscles to work harder for fast, effective body transformation.
Slim Series®	Debbie Siebers	60+ minutes	Advanced body slimming and toning focused on abs, thighs, butt, and hips.	Combines intense cardio with greater resistance to continue slimming and toning your body.

Cardio / Fat Burning Programs

Program Name	Trainer	Workout Duration	Benefits	How It Works
INSANITY®	Shaun T	30–60 minutes	Transform your body in 60 days with the most intense workout program ever put on DVD.	MAX Interval Training—you perform long bursts of maximum-intensity exercise with short periods of rest.
Turbo Jam®	Chalene Johnson	20–45 minutes	Calorie burning and total-body sculpting focused on abs and thighs.	Kickboxing and body sculpting to the hottest tunes to burn more calories than almost any other exercise.
Power 90®	Tony Horton	35–45 minutes	Fat burning and total-body sculpting focused on abs, thighs, and upper body.	90-day boot camp featuring fast and effective circuit-training workouts to transform your body in as little as 35 minutes a day.
Hip Hop Abs®	Shaun T	25–45 minutes	Calorie-burning cardio and total-body sculpting focused on abs and core.	Fun hip hop dance moves set to hot music to burn fat and sculpt lean sexy abs.
Brazil Butt Lift®	Leandro Carvalho	30–50 minutes	Reduce your hips, slim your thighs and lift your butt while you burn fat and melt away saddlebags.	Combines Brazilian dance, cardio, and signature sculpting moves with Leandro's proven TriAngle Training method that works your butt from multiple angles.
RevAbs™	Brett Hoebel	15–45 minutes	Fat-burning cardio, muscle-building and sculpting focused on abs and core.	Abcentrics™, Capoeira, cardio intervals, strength training, and ab/core work to get you six-pack abs in 90 days.
P90X® Plus	Tony Horton	20–45 minutes	The next level of advanced total-body training to get you ripped beyond belief.	Intense new cardio, muscle chiseling, and ab-/core-ripping moves to incorporate with P90X to ramp up your results.
Rockin' Body®	Shaun T	15–45 minutes	Calorie-burning cardio and full-body sculpting moves.	Party off the pounds as you dance and sweat to the hottest hits of all time.
Turbo Jam® Fat Burning Elite	Chalene Johnson	30–50 minutes	Advanced kickboxing and body-sculpting moves focused on core, thighs, and upper body.	More intense targeted workouts to maximize your fat-burning and sculpting results.

Abs/Core Programs

Program Name	Trainer	Workout Duration	Benefits	How It Works
RevAbs™	Brett Hoebel	15–45 minutes	Fat-burning cardio, muscle-building and sculpting focused on abs and core.	Abcentrics™, Capoeira, cardio intervals, strength training, and ab/core work to get you six-pack abs in 90 days.
Hip Hop Abs®	Shaun T	25–45 minutes	Calorie-burning cardio and total-body sculpting focused on abs and core.	Fun hip hop dance moves set to hot music to burn fat and sculpt lean sexy abs.
Turbo Jam®	Chalene Johnson	20–45 minutes	Calorie burning and total-body sculpting focused on abs and thighs.	Kickboxing and body sculpting to the hottest tunes to burn more calories than almost any other exercise.
P90X®	Tony Horton	45–60 minutes	Advanced total-body training program focused on abs, legs, chest, back, and arms.	Twelve routines that keep introducing new moves and challenging your muscles to get you absolutely ripped in 90 days.
Power 90®	Tony Horton	35–45 minutes	Fat burning and total-body sculpting focused on abs, thighs, and upper body.	90-day boot camp featuring fast and effective circuit-training workouts to transform your body in as little as 35 minutes a day.
Yoga Booty Ballet® Ab & Butt Makeover	Gillian Marloth and Teigh McDonough	35 minutes	Calorie burning and full-body sculpting focused on abs and booty.	Combines ab-sculpting yoga, booty-lifting ballet, and fat-melting cardio for total-body results while targeting your core and lower body.
Yoga Booty Ballet® Master Series	Gillian Marloth and Teigh McDonough	20–35 minutes	Advanced sculpting workouts focused on abs, thighs, and booty.	Yoga and Pilates moves designed to target your abs and booty in special workouts for any time of day.
Great Body Guaranteed!™	Tony Horton Debbie Siebers	under 10 minutes	Targeted body shaping focused on abs, arms, buns, and thighs.	Each move targets a specific zone to tighten and tone in under 10 minutes a day.

Dance Programs

Program Name	Trainer	Workout Duration	Benefits	How It Works
Hip Hop Abs®	Shaun T	25–45 minutes	Calorie-burning cardio and total-body sculpting focused on abs and core.	Fun hip hop dance moves set to hot music to burn fat and sculpt lean sexy abs. -
Shaun T's Dance Party Series™	Shaun T	30–40 minutes	Calorie-burning cardio and body-sculpting moves targeting abs and core.	Hot new dance moves and all-new music provide even more fun and challenging ways to party off the pounds and inches.
Hip Hop Abs® Ultimate Results	Shaun T	30–45 minutes	Advanced cardio and body-sculpting moves targeting abs and core.	High-energy dance moves set to hip hop music for cardio, strength, and advanced ab sculpting.
Rockin' Body®	Shaun T	15–45 minutes	Calorie-burning cardio and full-body sculpting moves.	Party off the pounds as you dance and sweat to the hottest hits of all time.
Brazil Butt Lift®	Leandro Carvalho	30–50 minutes	Reduce your hips, slim your thighs and lift your butt while you burn fat and melt away saddlebags.	Combines Brazilian dance, cardio, and signature sculpting moves with Leandro's proven TriAngle Training method that works your butt from multiple angles.
Yoga Booty Ballet® Ab & Butt Makeover	Gillian Marloth and Teigh McDonough	35 minutes	Calorie burning and full-body sculpting focused on abs and booty.	Combines ab-sculpting yoga, booty-lifting ballet, and fat-melting cardio for total-body results while targeting your core and lower body.
Turbo Jam® LIVE!	Chalene Johnson	30 minutes	Calorie burning and targeted body toning focused on abs and booty.	Live classes with fun dance-party feel for slimming and sculpting and rockin' results

Visit www.livingonhighspeed.com to learn more about these amazing workout programs.

All of these workout programs have been created by and are owned by Beach Body LLC.

Part 6

High Speed Tips

Chapter 10

High Speed Tips and Pointers

High Speed Blender (HSB) Tips

Over the last few years I have discovered that most HSBs are being under-utilized. Many people have told me they do not use their HSB enough. They often ask, "Can you give me a few tips on how to use my machine?"

Thus the Blender Tips section was created. These tips answer some of the questions I have been asked over the last few years. I trust these should simplify your daily High Speed Living journey.

Cleaning Your Machine

Remember you will never need to remove your HSB blades. Simply add to the container about 2 cups of water and 1 drop of dishwashing liquid, secure the lid and spin on high speed for a few seconds. Rinse and dry.

Occasionally you will need to wash your canister with a cloth and disinfectant of your choice. Placing your canister in the dishwasher is not recommended. But if you do, please remember to turn OFF the "high heat" dry cycle.

Placing Fruits / Vegetables In Your Machine

In any blending machine it is best to place liquids and softer items at the bottom of the container. HSBs are no exception.

But HSB machines do have advantages over all other blending devices.
- Vitamix owners have the advantage of the "Tamper". The Vitamix "Tamper" can be used to push stuck elements into the blades. With this tamper you can place whole fruits / vegetables in any order you like. But it will still be easier if you place softer items towards the bottom.

- Blendtec owners have the advantage of a wider base and larger blades. This wider base allows more fruit / vegetables to be blended without the need of a tamper device. Whole fruits and vegetables can be difficult to blend to total smoothness even in a Blendtec machine.

I have found that with both of these HSB machines if you place any fruits / vegetables into the containers properly you may never need to use a spoon or tamper again. This trick comes with time and practice.

Skins: Which Ones To Leave On And Which To Take Off

As a general rule most skins should / could be left intact. Why; because there are important nutrients in the skins of your fruits and vegetables. That being stated not all skins taste so good so here is the general guideline for determining to peel or not to peel.

The first rule I apply when leaving skins in-tact is to ensure you are using organic produce. And the second rule is to make sure your produce is clean. Lastly, remove the skins if you don't like the taste.

- Banana - NO – Nasty flavor
- Orange, grapefruit, tangerines - mostly no - very bitter
- Lemons / Limes - I leave them on most of the time, - pink lemonade, lime sorbet etc.
    - Lemon ice I take off the lemon zest
- Melons - Most are okay, just remember melon rinds can change the flavor.
    - I do not recommend cantaloupe melon rinds because fungus and molds concentrate in cantaloupe rinds more than other melons.
- Pomegranates – Remove the outer husk, leave the inner meat
- Garlic - Yes
- Onion - Yes

Froth Development – Why and What To Do

Unfortunately froth is going to develop. Not all fruits and veggies froth. But those that do, froth because of oxidation.

Here is what I recommend when froth appears. After the high speed blending cycle ends reduce the power level until the juice / smoothie forms a whirlpool in the center. This will pull everything from the top down to the bottom. Re-circulate the froth through the entire drink.

How Long Can Juices and Smoothies Be Stored

Research indicates that the nutrients in fruits and vegetables start to deplete or denature within twenty minutes. This does not mean that all nutrients deplete within that time but it does mean that you do not get 100%. So our primary recommendation is to enjoy your freshly blended drink immediately.

If you do store your drink for longer than twenty minutes, you may find that it will begin to separate. When separation occurs simply re-stir it or pour your drink back into your machine and spin on low speed.

Why Does My HSB Make Different Sounds?

From time to time you will hear different sounds coming from your HSB machine. In-fact sometimes it may seem that your machine has a life of its own! Be calm and learn to embrace your machine and it will give you great pleasure for many years to come.

Here is the breakdown of the sounds:
- High pitch scream – Your HSB has an air pocket, otherwise known as a hungry "empty" stomach. To fix this simply fill the empty tummy by pushing something into the void. If you own a Vitamix then you can use your tamper. When the air pocket has been filled, your HSB will stop screaming at you. Occasionally the noise will reoccur, especially when making ice cream or sorbets. No worries. Just fill the void again.
- Low pitch growl - This sound usually scares people. But it indicates something wonderful and delicious is being made. A HSB will "growl" at you when it has grabbed all of the elements and is doing a great job at churning your elements into nut butters, hummus, ice cream, sorbet, nut butters, fondues, hummus and other frozen or thick mixtures. Let it growl, 30 to 90 seconds usually this is all the time you will need to create something delicious and wonderful.
- Normal loud whirr - This is your machine humming along on high speed doing its job with normal elements like juices and smoothies. Life is good.

How Long Should I Spin My Elements

Desired consistency, determines spin time. Here are the guidelines I follow.
- Nut butters - 90 to 120 seconds with a lot of tamper usage.
- Hummus - 60 to 120 seconds
- Juice – Depending on the fruit or veggies involved. Usually anywhere from 60 seconds to 2 minutes. For instance hard elements like carrots take a full 2 minutes but bananas only take about 40 to 60 seconds.
  - Remember heat is being generated as you spin. Thus use ice or frozen elements to keep your juice cool during the spinning process.
- Smoothies – Apply the same guidelines as above while keeping the following in mind.
  - Hard seeds or heavily seeded items such as raspberries, seeded grapes, blackberries, pomegranates need more time to liquefy. Spin these element 90 seconds to 3 minutes.

Avoiding Common Raw / Vegan Mistakes

- Variety is the spice of life. Eating the same foods repeatedly leads to nutrient deficiencies.
- Keep it simple! Recipes that are complicated or have too many ingredients can keep new health enthusiast from becoming their best.
- Balancing Alkalinity. Stomach acid can become diluted or weak. This leads to gas, bloating, indigestion and other digestive issues. Follow my alkalinity steps in chapter 12.
- "Pull" the sweet tooth! Too many SWEET desserts (even raw desserts) can cause insulin and acidity problems. This includes all raw items such as chocolate, cheesecake, cookies, cakes, parfaits.
- It's not easy being green. Too much fruit and too few vegetables can cause nutritional imbalances! Leafy greens should comprise half of your diet!
- Be simply raw. This is yet another old world habit to be broken. We want our "junk" foods. So we dehydrate to make the "raw" taste and feel like our old comfort foods (crackers, cereal, breads, kale chips, fruit roll ups, candied nuts and more!) Become a simple raw foodist!

- Detox and be free flowing! Get clean by performing normal detox programs and occasional enemas and colonics to help detox your body on a regular basis.
- Get to the root of the problem. Roots are the mainstay of most vegans and raw foodies. Roots are harder to digest, contain less nutrients and have far more sugar than the leafy green counterparts. Eat carrot tops instead of the carrot root.
- Chew your food! Most Americans do not chew their food properly. Undigested cellulose causes gas, malnutrition, over-eating and other associated digestive disorders. Chew your food twenty to thirty times before swallowing.
- Move your body! Many raw, vegan and vegetarians that I have met believe they are healthy and do not need to "workout". But there is hard evidence showing that cardio and weight bearing exercises are necessities to creating total wellness.
- Food combining. Each food type requires different digestion times. Meats and processed foods take the longest to digest and nuts and root vegetables take longer than fruit. All food stays in the stomach during the entire digestion process so fruits will sit in your stomach while harder to digest items are being dissolved. Gas, bloating and other digestive issues can occur! Eat fruit separate from other foods.
- Get soaked! Raw nuts and seeds have growth inhibitors that make them tough and keeps them from sprouting prematurely. Soaking will remove this inhibitor enzyme making it easier on your body's digestion and absorption system.
- Going nuts! Don't go nuts. Eat more seeds. They are better for you!
- Eat early. Eat before the sun goes down and your body will not have to work as hard overnight.
- "Pull" that other sweet tooth. Using incorrect sweeteners like agave nectar, aspartame, sweet-n-low, splenda and more is bad news. Latest findings show us that these items are not good for you and can keep you from losing weight and detoxing properly.
- Relax and de-stress! Staying in a stressed state can cause many known and unknown illness issues.
- Cheating to win? Most people cheat more than they think. Keep a food log for a while and you would be surprised!
- Get essential! Get all of the essential elements into your body. Things like seaweed, MSM, blue green algaes and other superfoods contain elements

that are not in other food sources and these elements are vital. So get some!

- Enzymes, enzymes, enzymes! Sensing a theme about digestion being important?
- Get Your Protein. Protein and amino acids are the building blocks of your cells! You need protein to maintain and build muscle and tissue! If you have opted to not consume meat, you can still obtain adequate amounts of protein with the following:
    - **Sprouts** – Sprouts provide a good source of protein. Sprouts take less time to digest than meat. Sprouts are living food, meat is lifeless. Sprouts are alkaline, meat is acidic. Sprouts can reduce grocery cost, meat is a highly priced. Sprouts have no additives, meat may have hormones and chemicals. Sprouts have zero cholesterol.
    - **Dark Leafy Greens** – Green leafy vegetables, when eaten raw, are a great source of amino acids - the building blocks of protein. They are easiest to digest and assimilate when well blended, juiced, or thoroughly chewed. Green smoothies are an increasingly popular way to get high quantities of greens into the diet on a daily basis. Rotate your greens weekly: Kale, Watercress, Arugula, Collard Greens, Broccoli, Brussel Sprouts, Spinach, Parsley
    - **Sea Vegetables** – Sea vegetables absorb nutrients from the ocean and are considered to be some of the most mineral rich foods on the planet. Most seaweeds are at least 50% protein based. This includes plants such as: Dulse, Nori, Kelp and Wakame.
    - **Grasses** – Grasses are a complete food. An analysis performed and provided by the Anne Wigmore Foundation showed 3500 mg. of wheat grass to contain the following protein count: 800 mg. This includes the following grass types: wheatgrass, barley and alfalfa.
    - **Algaes** – Algaes are considered to be the most complete food on the planet. In fact we now know that one could thrive on algae if there were no other foods. Protein content is as high as 64%. This includes the following algae types: chlorella, spirulina and blue green algae.
    - **Seeds** – Each seed varies on protein content but nearly all seeds contain all amino acids and are high in absorbable protein content. Chia seeds are roughly 18% to 22% protein and one Tbsp provide

2 to 4 grams of protein. Hemp seeds contain roughly 5 to 7 grams of protein per Tbsp. Also consider other soaked & sprouted seeds.

- o **Soaked Beans/Lentils/Legumes** – Beans are not the highest protein content in the plant kingdom but they are one of the most abundant, most widely used and well accepted alternative protein sources for vegans and raw foodist. Here are a few examples: Black beans – 8oz. = 15g protein, black eyed peas – 8oz. = 13g protein, kidney beans – 8oz. = 16g protein.

Remember to soak raw beans to remove the enzyme growth inhibitor.

- o **Soaked Grains** – Whole grains are a great source of protein. Quinoa is the king of grains with over 18g of protein for every 8oz but enjoy other soaked non cooked grains as well.
- o **Bee Pollen -** The protein content of bee pollen ranges from 10 to 35 percent (according to its plant origin). All pollens contain the exact same number of 22 amino acids, yet different species produce varying amounts. There is roughly 5g of protein for every 1 Tbsp of bee pollen.
- o **Brewers Yeast & Nutritional Yeast -** Nutritional yeast contains high levels of many important nutrients, including all of the B vitamins (except for B_{12}), 16 amino acids. Brewer's yeast has 4 to 5g per every 1 Tbsp, making it a rich source of protein for vegetarians.
- o **Plant Based Protein Powders** – A few select companies have created clean vegetarian protein powders (soy, pea, hemp, chia etc). Seek these out at one of your local health food stores.
- o **Soaked Nuts** – Nuts are great source of protein. They are tasty, easy to eat, and can be added into any meal, dessert, salad or smoothie. The downside is that nuts have more calories than seeds, they are harder for the body to digest and the oils can go rancid if stored improperly. Rancidity is bad for the body. It is also important to point out that nuts contain unsaturated fat which is a good fat (compared to saturated fat which is found in red meats).

The following protein content per nut type is based on a 3.5oz serving size:
Pecans, 9.5g – Peanuts, 24g – Almonds, 21g – Cashews, 18g, - Hazelnut, 15g

Time Saving Tips

Eating properly can be overwhelming in the beginning. So here are a few tips to help you through the transition.

- Use your high speed blender! It saves TIME!
- Plan your meals ahead of time.
- Prepare your meals ahead of time and freeze or refrigerate them for later use.
- Consume raw meal replacements. Meal replacements are usually loaded with great   nutrition and they are great time savers.
- Get freezer safe containers to store your food.
- Find foods that you like that you know are good for you and find an easy and quick way to prepare and store.
- Carry easy foods like hard boiled eggs, vegetables, fruits, and etc..

Cleaning Tips

Do you clean your produce and have you ever wondered whether those expensive veggie washes are worth the money?

Research by multiple organizations to include *"Cook's Illustrated"* and the Institute of Agricultural and Environmental Sciences at Tennessee State University indicates that your produce can have 98 percent of bacteria removed using proper cleaning techniques.

Each organization tested multiple techniques such as veggie washes, soapy water, pure water, brushing and vinegar solutions.
In the end the Vinegar solution beat out all other cleaning techniques and has shown to be effective to reduce bacteria levels by as much as 98 percent.

Cleaning with Vinegar

Make the cleaning solution of three (3) parts pure water to one (1) part vinegar. Place the solution in a spray bottle for an easy misting system to clean your plants.

A few squirts of the solution is enough to coat the surface of most fruit. Let sit for 30 or so seconds and then scrub with a soft brush and rinse under the tap.

This technique works best for smooth skinned fruits and vegetables. Textured items such as broccoli, lettuce leaves, kale or spinach prove to be much harder to clean.
For the deeply textured vegetables like broccoli or cauliflower that have lots of crevices I recommend filling a sink with the solution and soak the deeply textured items in the solution for a full two minutes.

Adding a tablespoon of baking soda is very effective for removing stubborn stuck on dirt and debris both when scrubbing leaves and other textured items.

In a pinch, some cleaning does occur if you simply "rub" your fruit on a clean cloth. But remember this tip: bacteria and dirt are usually trapped at the blossom and stem ends of fruit so make it a habit to slice off both ends after rinsing.

Food can become contaminated with harmful bacteria where it is produced, where it is sold, or even on your kitchen counter. Here are some tips on how to prevent food-borne illness:

Wash your hands often.

Yes, that age-old advice is still the best way to avoid getting sick. Use hot water and soap to wash your hands before and after handling food. 30 seconds or more of scrubbing under running water should do the trick.

Disinfect dishes, cutting boards and counters with hot, soapy water after preparing each food item.

Bacteria from one food item could remain on cutting boards, dishes or counters and contaminate the next food item prepared. A solution of one teaspoon of bleach in one quart of water can be used to sanitize all surfaces and utensils. For effective sanitation a bleach solution needs to sit on the surface for about 10 minutes. Vinegar also works well for those who prefer not to use bleach for either personal or environmental reasons.

Use special precautions for raw meat, poultry and seafood.

I know this is a Raw and Vegetarian preparation guide, but for those who occasionally do prepare meat for themselves, family or friends, please take care to keep raw meat, poultry and seafood separated from other foods. From the minute you take these raw meats from the store shelf until you cook them it is best to keep them in plastic bags to prevent juices from dripping onto surfaces or other foods. The uncooked juices can contain and spread harmful bacteria.

Use separate cutting boards for your raw meat. Don't use the same cutting boards for your fresh produce.

Marinate food in the refrigerator not on the counter.

Sauce used for marinating raw meat, poultry or seafood should never be reused on cooked food! After marinating the meat, TOSS the remaining marinated sauces.

Refrigerate or freeze leftovers within two hours of cooking.

Cool temperatures keep most harmful bacteria from multiplying. Store food in clean, covered containers.

Part 7

Living On High Speed

Chapter 11

A High Speed Road Map To Success

Finding a balance between living a modern fast paced life and maintaining great health can be a challenge. Many factors vie for your time. Things such as your profession, searching for work, school, personal hobbies, community and volunteer work, family/children are lifestyle choices that we each face. At times balancing a hectic lifestyle with a healthy lifestyle is even challenging for me. But with a little planning and can do attitude, balance can be achieved. In fact, millions have already found balance and are living vibrant and healthy lives. I believe that you also can achieve balance if you are ready for a change and are willing to accept the information and tips that I and many other wellness educators provide.

Over the years I have helped many people to achieve their goals either for health and fitness or balanced lifestyles. I found the following guidelines to be the most successful tips in helping them to achieve their dreams. I believe these steps will also help you!

To help guide you through your personal wellness journey I have broken this section into two parts.

1. **Decide, Commit, Modify** – This is your guide to continuous success. Follow this protocol and apply it to your life week after week and you will find success in your life.
2. **Steps To Living A High Speed Life** – These are the wellness steps I have given to hundreds of people and the same steps I use to maintain a healthy lifestyle. To help you further understand how to use this section I have broken this into three parts.
    i.   Change Your Body
    ii. Change Your Mind
    iii. Change Your Energy

If you would like to mold these steps into your current lifestyle and form them into a working plan that fits you, then join hundreds of other like-minded people online at www.livingonhighspeed.com and become a member of the life changing **Vortex Zone**.

Decide, Commit, Modify

1) Decide

  a) Decide to live a purpose filled life at a higher energy level. Decide to make a change for the better. Decide to make changes that will improve the quality of life for you and for the world around you.

  b) Decide on a road map to get you to that higher level of living. This should include setting your goals, creating a properly balanced living foods meal plan and a spiritual/mental/physical workout plan that will fit **YOU.** Finding the proper fit for your lifestyle is crucial to your success.

2) Commit

  a) Commit to your plan and stick with it.

  b) Commit to a success partner / mentor / accountability partner.

  c) Commit to announcing your new journey and tell the world – The more people who know your intentions the harder it is to give up on your goals quietly.

  d) Commit to tracking your goals.

   Take before pictures & measurements.

3) Modify

  a) Continually listen to your inner voice. Pay attention to how your body feels. Continually modify your Road Map based on what that inner voice is telling you and watch how your body is responding.

   I am not talking about that self defeating voice. The one we call the ego. Instead tap into your inner spiritual consciousness.

  b) Modify your goals, your workouts, eating plans and your spiritual walk as needed until you find the proper path that fits you. Then repeat steps 1 and 2.

Sometimes our bodies and minds need a little different motivation and stimulation than originally anticipated. If this is the case, be patient and listen to your body and your mind. Make a few adjustments and always keep moving forward.

One final note on succeeding; every day people fail to meet their goals for many reasons. Lack of internal desire, personal commitment and goal setting are usually the main reasons for failure no matter what the endeavor. Most people, even coaches and personal trainers, cannot help you with creating more internal passion. But these professionals and possibly even your friends can definitely help you with maintaining your personal commitment and sticking to your goals.

That being stated, I want you to re-read these most over looked success factors:
Commit to your plan and stick with it.
Commit to a success partner / mentor / accountability partner.
Commit to announcing your new journey and tell the world – The more people who know your intentions the harder it is to give up on your goals quietly.
Commit to tracking your goals.

The bottom line is this: Tell the world, set your goals and FIND someone with whom you feel comfortable who will push you to become successful and minimize your exposure to those who are a negative influence.

Your success partners can be anyone! They do not necessarily need to be with you during your workouts or at your home when you are updating your goals and eating your meals. (Though having someone close to you is optimal.) Partners can keep you inspired when you are down, pick you up when you drag, point out when your form is not correct, keep you from sand bagging a workout, keep you from cheating on your diet, keep you from missing a day and so much more.

I have found that even being aware that a few extra people were in the gym kept me on top of my form. This was mental of course because my ego wants to look good in front of others. But it worked and it kept me from slouching and I felt myself reaching for that extra centimeter when perhaps I would not have done so without an on-looker.

So in short, find someone that wants to see you succeed as much as you do and stick with them!

NOTE: I have put together an amazing accountability program called the "Vortex Zone". The "Vortex Zone" is your answer to connecting with me and other likeminded people who are all willing to hold each other accountable to achieving their best. We will host daily and weekly motivational video and blog updates, weekly and monthly goal setting meetings, weekly conference calls, amazing video recipes, health tips and advice from Vortex members and much more! Go to www.livingonhighspeed.com to join the Vortex Zone today!

Chapter 12

Steps To Living Your High Speed Life

The definition of a vortex is a whirling or rotary motion of a liquid, gas, flame, wind and etc that sucks everything towards its center. In the vortex of a hurricane, tornado or even your HSB there is an eerie yet awe-inspiring calm. Everything in the calm is protected and charged with energy while everything outside of this calm is whirling at high speed creating this energy.

Additionally, while high speed blenders cannot top the speed of an F5 tornado, they do come close. The top speed of an F5 tornado is 318 mph. The top speed of commercial high speed machines range between 240 to 300 mph. If you know anything about an F5 then you know this, there is not a force in nature that can stop an F5. And if you know your high speed blenders then you know this, there is not a fruit, vegetable, herb, wild or domesticated plant or superfood that can stop your HSB.

Likewise when you are living on high speed and living within the vortex your life energy is aligned with universal energies that will quickly bring many awesome things into your life like greater happiness, more love and generosity, new friends and business associates, greater success in all endeavors and in some cases even more prosperity.

My wish for you is to: live on high speed, use your high speed blenders, live with purpose and redirect and change your energy to establish a new vortex and "pull-in" successful energy and successful people. And above all expunge the negative energy and the negative toxins that are in your body and in your mind.

The following steps have been extracted from my life changing "Vortex Plan". The Vortex Plan was created to help you live on high speed. I have applied these concepts to my own life and achieved great success. I believe if you apply these concepts to your life, you will achieve your personal goals.

The steps are arranged and sorted by the same motto I use to excite people to change their lives.

Change Your Body / Change Your Mind / Change Your Life Energy

Some of these steps are complex and take a lifetime to master while others may take just a few days. All separately and all together are a process.

So, add a few steps each week, one each day or as fast or slow as needed in your life. Just decide to make that change and stay true and committed to it and you should start noticing a positive difference in your physical, mental and spiritual wellbeing.

Remember: Success is not a destination, it is a journey.

* **IMPORTANT** * Always apply and follow the DECIDE – COMITT – MODIFY protocols as you journey through the steps in this chapter. It will be much easier to succeed if you do.

By the way, make sure you visit my website www.livingonhighspeed.com and join the Vortex Zone to learn more about the following exciting challenge program:
- Living On High Speed 1 Year Change Your Life Challenge

Change Your Body

Out of the three phases:
1. Change Your Body
2. Change Your Mind
3. Change Your Energy

I find that changing your body is the easiest. Changing old mind sets, disarming hot buttons and achieving spiritual oneness are a little more difficult to master.

Step 1: Use Your High Speed Blenders (HSB) Daily

For generations health advocates and nutrition counselors have been using HSBs and juice extractors to create amazing life giving meals.

When you use your HSB daily you will join the ranks of thousands who have transformed their lives by discovering the power of raw living foods.

The more often you ingest liquid living foods, the more easily your body will become detoxified and your body will more easily remove body fat and restore your inner health.

Example- blended meals I make:
- Fresh fruit and vegetable smoothie
  - Use the blending chart or the recipes in the recipes section for some delicious ideas.
  - Avoid fruit if you are trying to reduce your fat stores quickly.
  - Feel free to add one or two superfoods as listed in the "Superfoods" section in part 2 of this book.
- Leafy greens juice
  - The darker the greens the better. (i.e. kale, collard greens, mustard greens, spinach, carrot top greens, beet top greens and etc.)
  - Feel free to add one or two superfoods as listed in the "Superfoods" section in part 2 of this book.
  - Use the blending chart listed at the beginning of the recipe section for a few delicious ideas.
- Superfood elixirs
  - Pure superfood drink using fresh young coconut water or some other raw superfood liquid.
  - Add the daily superfoods and a few of the other supperfoods to create something delicious and life giving.

Step 2: Use The "Daily" SuperFoods Daily

Add the "daily" superfoods (found in chapter 6) to your blended drinks, normal meals or eat them straight up. It does not matter as long as you add them to your daily routine!
See the "Superfoods" section to learn more about each superfood I recommend.
- Also remember to use any other SuperFoods as often as possible.

Step 3: Sprout And Have No Doubt

Sprouts contain all elements a plant needs for life and growth. These same elements are in large part what your body needs to repair and rebuild those 60 trillion cells that split inside of you on a daily basis. When you sprout your seeds they germinate. Germination converts starch to simple sugar, causes fat to break down into life giving EFAs, minerals merge with protein thus increasing digestible nutrient content and proteins become predigested amino acids. Research shows that sprouts contain one of the highest rated vitamin and mineral content.

Among their other virtues sprouted seeds are low in cost, can be stored indefinitely, are easy to grow, and when sprouted increase their nutritional value many times.

Sprouts are best when eaten raw. You can eat the entire sprout, including leaves and roots. Sprouts can be eaten by themselves, be added to salads, sandwiches, soups, blended for smoothies, baby food, sauces, and dressings. They can be stored for up to two weeks if refrigerated.

Other Attributes Of Sprouting
- Sprouts are a powerful source of antioxidants in the form of vitamins, minerals and enzymes which assist in protecting the body from free radical damage.
- Sprouts are alkaline.
- Sprouts are full of living enzymes.
- Sprouts can be grown in your kitchen.
- Sprouts are a good source of essential fatty acids (EFA).
- Sprouts are high in fiber.
- Sprouts have a massive supply of vitamins. Research suggest that the vitamin content of some seeds can increase from 100% to 2000% in several days of sprouting.
- Sprouts are high in minerals. During sprouting, the minerals are enriched and chelation occurs making these minerals easier to be absorbed in your body.
- Sprouts can be grown all year round to give a constant supply of food in the very freshest form possible.
- Sprouts provide a good source of protein. Sprouts take less time to digest than meat, sprouts are living food - meat is lifeless, sprouts are alkaline -

meat is acidic, sprouts can cut the cost of living - meat is a highly priced, sprouts have no additives - meat may have hormones and chemicals from farming practices, sprouts have zero cholesterol.
- Sprouts are low in calories.
- Sprouts have a low glycemic index.
- Sprouts are awesome nutrient-dense foods.

How to Sprout

SEEDS – Soak about one to two tablespoonfuls (seeds will expand about eight times the original amount) in a large glass jar. Fill the jar half-way with tepid water and cover it with something that breathes like cheese-cloth. Secure the cloth with a rubber band. Place in a dark area at about room temperature for about five hours. After five hours, drain, rinse, and let the seeds stand without water for about eight to twelve hours. Rinse again and drain well to prevent rotting. For the next six days the seeds should be rinsed and drained twice a day using lukewarm water. They should be kept at room temperature in a dark place. After the sixth day, place them in the light for one more day to increase their chlorophyll content.

GRAINS – Preparation is the same as for seeds.

LEGUMES – Due to their hardness, legumes and beans can require an initial soaking of about fifteen hours. They should be rinsed twice a day and given three days for adequate sprouting. Legume expansion is not so great as in the case of seeds and grains.

Step 4: Avoid the "Top Foods Not to Eat" And Consume Living Foods

Mentor, educator and Director of the Hippocrates Health Institute Brian Clement stated the following at a raw food expo "We have to be crazy to think processed food is what we should be eating." At least that is what I remember him saying.

The bottom line is this: **Don't Eat Processed Foods!**

Processed foods do not provide life giving nutrients and are in most cases considered to be dangerous for your body. All processed foods should be avoided but focusing on removing the following list from your diet will help ensure your goals will be met in a timely manner. Additionally, as you add more raw living foods and remove more of the foods listed below the more energy and life will be given back to your body.

1. Pork, high fat luncheon meats, ham, pepperoni, hot dogs, bacon and sausage meat.
2. Shellfish: oysters, scallops, clams, crab, and lobster. They are scavengers and feed off the bottom of the ocean. Also contain high levels of mercury.
3. Aspartame, Nutrasweet, Equal and most other artificial sweeteners.
4. Hydrogenated, partially hydrogenated oils or lard.
5. Junk Food: snack cakes, candy, cola, fast food, pizza etc.
6. Dairy products: milk, cheese, creams, yogurts and other bovine produced milk elements.
7. Chlorinated water. Chlorine is a deadly toxin. "Either use a filter or become a filter"!
8. Alcohol: Just 1 oz of alcohol reduces the body's ability to burn fat by 30%.
9. Pasta & Breads: the only breads I recommend are sprouted grain products like Ezekiel.
10. And the last but one of the most important items to remove from your diet is all **fried food**! Heated and superheated oil is DANGEROUS. Research shows us that oils degrade easily to toxic compounds and release dangerous free radicals when heated. And it has been shown that prolonged consumption of burnt oils lead to atherosclerosis, inflammatory joint disease, development of birth defects and a host of other inflammatory diseases.

Now this list may seem daunting. More than a few people have told me in exasperation "This is everything I currently eat. What am I supposed to eat instead?"

By now you should know the answer to this. Yes you guessed right. Replace the above items with raw living foods. I would like to see each of you to become a 100% living food enthusiast. But if you are new to this concept then switching to a 100% living foods diet may be a little tough. So eat as much living foods as possible every day. Try to shoot for at least 70% to 80% living food consumption.

Remember that the green leafy foods contain the most nutrients. Vegetables and herbs are next. Fruits are last. While this book contains blended meals, I will ensure my second book will contain many normal, non-blended recipes.

You may not be able to switch out all of your poor quality foods for high quality foods in one week or even one month but this is an important step. Make small changes every single day. Add new and exciting veggies and fruits every few days and make this new journey a fun one.

In a few months you will be a new person!

Read the end of this book and my www.livingonhighspeed.com web site to see an exciting challenge I have put together to help you achieve your goals!

Step 5: Eat 5 or 6 Small Meals Through Out the Day

There is overwhelming evidence that eating multiple times throughout the day can greatly improve your health. The below points highlight just a few of the reasons you may want to try this. Now don't get me wrong, you cannot eat Twinkies and Ding Dongs six times a day. Nor should you be eating processed foods, refined sugars or flour. Stick to eating life giving vegetables, fruits, herbs and other superfoods at least 70% to 80% of the time and your life will forever be changed.

If you do eat meat products then remember to enjoy range fed meats and wild caught fish. Farm raised animals have been subjected to far too many unhealthy living conditions to be advantageous for your body. Also remember that you can obtain more bio-available proteins from algae, dark leafy greens and from other sources like hemp seed and chia seeds.

Reasons To Eat 5 or 6 Meals Each Day

- Speeds up metabolism.
- Long term consumption of hard to digest large meals that are poor nutrient dense meals causes your body to "shut" down and hibernate. When this occurs the body stores more of your consumed meals as fat and stores toxins that are hidden inside of the processed foods you consume inside of your fat tissue.
- Diminishes the desire to overeat.
- Puts less stress on your colon.

- Easier for your body to digest.
- Stabilize blood sugar levels.

Eating 5 to 6 small meals everyday can be more easily achieved if you add the following two factors to your lifestyle.
1. Using Your HSB
   - Blended meals are easier for your body to digest.
   - Liquid and blended meals help to detox your body quicker than solid meals.
   - The more blended meals you enjoy the faster you will see results like weight loss and disease management.
   - Blended meals are much quicker to prepare than conventional meals.
   - Blended meals are easier to cleanup.
   - Enjoy at least one if not two or more per day. The more you do, again the quicker you will see amazing results

2. Meal Replacement Supplements
   In a perfect world we would not need "supplements". After all "supplements" are designed to do just what the name states, "supplement" your daily dietary consumption in order to provide the required amount of life giving nutrients that your body needs to survive and sometimes even to improve your performance or your results.

   But sadly our world is far from perfect. In fact I believe that many things in our world have been turned upside down. With over 66% of America being overweight, I think there is NO refuting these statements: "Fast food, processed food, microwaves, pesticide infested farms, man-made chemicals to make products addictive, tainted livestock, meat and dairy farms, legislation to keep you from growing your own organic foods and many more things have been forced onto us by big business and government. This has resulted in an overweight yet under-nourished nation.

   So what are we to do? First we should do our best to avoid all man-made processed food. Then do our best to eat clean organic foods and support local farmers and not support big tycoon food manufactures. And then add organic, raw, living foods to our daily dietary consumption.

Know the following about supplementation:

- It is near impossible to obtain all the vitamins, enzymes, minerals and phytonutrients we need from our processed foods and even from your fruits and vegetables. Food is depleted because the soil is depleted. Remember your bodies are comprised of vitamins and minerals which you need to re-supply constantly.
- Not all supplements are created equal so do your research before purchasing.
- Not all supplements are for all people. Each supplement typically has a targeted purpose. Creatine and protein help build muscle while pyruvate stabilizes blood sugar levels. Do your home work!

I have a few favorites when it comes to using supplements.

- For instance I love all superfoods as long as they have not been processed and overheated.
- I enjoy sports supplements like creatine occasionally. (I always need to detox after using them for extended periods.)
- And I enjoy a product called Shakeology.
    - Shakeology is often touted as being the "One supplement to rule them all"!
    - Shakeology combines 70 of the worlds known superfoods in one delicious drink. This way you do not have to search the world over for all of the superfoods.
        - Shakeology can help you:
            a. Lose Weight
            b. Feel Energized
            c. Improve Digestion and Regularity
            d. Lower Cholesterol

Find where I get my supplements at www.livingonhighspeed.com

Step 6: Detox And Cleanse Your Body

Have you ever marveled at the complexity of the human body? It is a fine-tuned, complex machine similar to yet much more complex than a high performance sports car. So, if it makes sense to perform normal maintenance on your car (changing the oil, the tires, the spark plugs, cleaning the fuel injection system, changing the belts, cleaning the interior and the exterior), then shouldn't it also make sense to also perform regular maintenance on your body?

Regular auto maintenance and clean fuel ensures peak performance and lengthens the life of your automobile. Changing the oil means removing old dirty oil and infusing your car with fresh clean oil. This simple act keeps your engine running smoother and longer and decreases repair cost.

In today's fast paced world people find the time to perform basic maintenance on their cars. But most people fail to perform the same regular maintenance with their bodies. Does this seem strange to you? It does seem very strange to me.

So get to it! Start performing "normal maintenance" and feed your body with clean feul, detox your body and enjoy a healthier happier life.

There are many ways to detox and hundreds of cleansing programs available to you: liver cleanse, colon cleanse, water cleanse, juice cleanse, fasting, heavy metal cleanse, parasite cleanse, master cleanse, coffee enemas, wheatgrass enemas and many more some of which work and are effective and some that are slightly dangerous. Some detoxification programs can be purchased in a kit form: "Perfect Cleanse", "Ultimate Cleanse", "Super Colon Cleanse" and many more.

Whichever cleanse you select, just do it. I find it is best to perform small cleanses throughout the year and perform deep cleanses at least twice a year.

The longer the cleanse/detox session the better things will be for your body. But typically after the first week of an intense cleanses the worse you will likely feel. Some people refer to this as a "healing crisis" because you may start to look like you are sick at some point. This happens because your body is releasing toxins. When toxins are released strange side effects may occur. Because of this your friends may think you are crazy and they may try to stop you from cleansing. But if you stick it out, you will be pleasantly surprised with the benefits.

Here is an example general cleanse many people have followed. If you wish further cleanse instruction or targeted cleanse protocols, contact me and I will provide the specific details.

- Enjoy 5 to 7, eight ounce glasses of vegetable juice every day for five to seven days (or longer if you can).
- Enjoy two high speed blended drinks per day during the same time period.
- Drink only pH balanced purified water during this time.
- Do not ingest any solid food during this cleanse period.
- Leafy green vegetables are the most nutrient dense.

At the end of this protocol I suggest that you ease back into eating solid food. Follow something similar to the following for the following week.

- Enjoy one to two high speed blended vegetable only drinks per day for at least five to seven days or longer as desired.
- Enjoy two to three high speed blended 1 fruit / 2 vegetable drinks per day during the same period.
- Enjoy one serving of fresh fruit and two fresh vegetable salads each day during the same period.

After this two week period, try your best to ingest only a living foods diet for an additional two weeks.

I guarantee this will change your life!

Step 7: Drink Water

Most people do not drink enough water. They think they do but most Americans are severely dehydrated and disease bound due to low water intake. Consuming too little fresh pure water is one of the many contributing factors towards becoming very unhealthy. To make matters worse, most people assume that the fluids that they do drink contribute to their daily water requirements. But the opposite is true. Many drinks like coffee, alcohol and carbonated beverages are diuretic in nature. Diuretics cause cells to quickly lose body fluid. Other drinks are loaded with sugars and chemical compounds. These toxic substances clog your filtering systems and cause a backlog of toxin buildup inside of your fat and tissue cells.

Besides drinking toxic substances like carbonated beverages, coffee and alcohol there are other associated problems to consider.

1) Tap water is TOXIC - There are way too many chemicals (chemicals kill living things) in our public water supply to consider it a healthy resource. Note: Tap water is still not as detrimental to the human body as a soda drink. So stay away from carbonate soft drinks!!!

2) Most bottle water is also tap water – The secret is out. Research has revealed that large corporations are passing off bottled tap water as filtered healthy water. Filtering systems are expensive and many large corporations are not investing in them.

So the moral of this story: Buy a good filter system for your home. Remember this, "Use a filter or become one".

- Drink at least half your body weight in ounces per day of filtered, pure pH balanced water. Example a 100 lbs female needs at least 50oz. of water and a 200 lbs man needs at least 100 oz. of filtered water each day.
- The easiest way to remember / track your water intake is to purchase a container the size of your minimum daily requirement of water that you need. Fill the container at the beginning of each morning and drink from the container throughout the day. Make sure it is empty by the end of the day.
- Remember you need over 5 to 7 glasses of water to compensate for 1 soda. So, if you drink any diuretics you must drink more water to compensate your lost body fluids.
- Water helps balance your pH.
- Water helps removes toxins and debris from your body.
- Research shows when we are born our body is 85% water but when we die our body is about 50% water.
- Drink your water 10 to 15 minutes before a meal and avoid drinking during the meal. And drink your water 15 to 30 minutes after a fruit / veggie meal and about 1 hour after a hard to digest meal like meats or processed foods.

This dehydration is avoidable and is up to you.

When you drink water, toxins are swept away, your blood becomes thinned, nutrients are carried and absorbed more easily, your cells heal easier and many more amazing things happen. You will feel better if you hydrate yourself.

For better absorption and to improve alkalinity add the following elements to your water: pinch sea salt, 1/8 tsp baking soda & 8 drops trace minerals.

Step 8: Consume a High Fiber Diet

I often see commercials encouraging people to eat a high fiber diet. Admittedly eating a high fiber diet is a good thing because fiber happens to be an important aspect of your wellness journey. But sadly, these commercials usually promote manmade fiber. These manmade fibers have been added to foods like cereals, crackers, fake fruit treats and other processed foods. These fiber enriched foods are typically void of nutrients yet high in calories. So what are we to do?

Modern societies typically eat a "non" fiber diet rich in meats, pasta, refined breads, sweet treats and other manmade or processed foods.

So where is the fiber? Real natural fiber is found within the live vegetables, fruits, herbs and unprocessed whole grains and legumes. So if you made any simple change to your diet I would recommend this:

Design your diet to be comprised of at least 70% or more of vegetable, fruits, legumes and unprocessed grains.

High fiber diets have the following benefits:
- Lower cholesterol levels.
- Decreases risk of colon cancer as much as 60%.
- Regulates the colon.
- Gives truth to the wise saying "an apple a day keeps the doctor away".
- Fiber fills you so one has the sensation of being "satiated" and will naturally stop eating.
- Levels insulin sugar spikes.

Tip: Use a high speed blender to make your fiber more bio-available!

Step 9: Essential Fats

Ahh fats... the good, the bad and the ugly. There have been volumes written on the subject of fats. But for the most part, FAT gets a bad rap. In fact, saturated fat (mostly stemming from animal products) has received most of the brunt of all of the bad press.

Although saturated fats can be unhealthy if not kept to a minimum, it is not saturated fats that are causing the majority of obesity and disease related health problems. The real issue is what happens to fat when it has been processed!

In general, research indicates that breads, cakes, cookies, crackers, cereals, pasta, chemical additives, flavor extracts, processed foods and the **BIG one, partially hydrogenated oils**, are more to blame for clogged arteries, blood issues and other blockages within the human body.

I recommend instead of eliminating all meats try to first discard ALL of your pre processed food items that are in your pantry! You will be much healthier and happier for it. If you opt to not join the living foods world then do your best to ingest smaller quantities of meat products a few times each month. Learn to enjoy wild caught fish which is less saturated with fats than beef. Make sure all animal products are range fed and organic fed.

Now there are some fats that are GOOD for you. They are called essential fatty acids or EFAs. These types of fats are used daily by the body to perform many vital functions. There are 2 ways to obtain EFA fats.
1) Plant sources: Like but not limited to - Flax, borage, primrose, hemp, chia and etc.
2) Fish sources: Specifically deep sea fish like but not limited to cod, mackerel, krill and etc.
Be aware that some research has shown that fish EFA's can go "rancid" and therefore can be harmful to the body.

My discussion here is not meant to be comprehensive in nature. Instead, go to Amazon or any local book store and you will find a large variety of books written about the subject of EFAs. Just be aware of claims like "this EFA Source is better than others" because in most cases writers / authors usually are slightly biased because they are selling a specific brand. Thus their article / book will be slanted towards that brand. Instead, start using any EFA and listen to your body.

If your body is responding well then stick with it for a while. And then add another brand at a later time to add some diversity to your diet. If your body has trouble adjusting to your current EFA, switch to a different brand or EFA source.

Here are just a few ways in which EFA's can help.
- Rebuild and produce new cells.
- Protects cell walls.
- Proper brain formation in infants and children.
- Elasticity of skin.
- Stabilize blood sugar levels if taken while eating.
- Destroys bad cholesterol in the body.
- Lubricate the body from the inside out so that you will not need lotion.

I use a few different EFAs sources on a daily basis. Udo's Choice, flax seeds, hemp seeds, chia seeds, krill and marine phytoplankton.

Step 10: Control Your Alkalinity

Within your body exists a natural "acid" base. This acid base is part of multiple processes that occur within your body. The human body auto regulates this base during certain stages. For instance, in the digestive system the stomach acid (pH) drops to 2 when you ingest food. Yet when this food exits your stomach your system creates bicarbonate to raise your pH to 7 thus protecting your intestines from being damaged by the stomach acid.

Alkalinity is important in other areas of your body such as the respiratory system and the metabolic system. Each process is very prone to change depending on many factors which will be discussed below. pH refers to "potential hydrogens" and is measured on a scale from 1 (very acidic) to 7 (neutral) to 14 (very alkaline).

"The countless names of illnesses do not really matter. What does matter is that they all come from the same root cause...too much tissue acid waste in the body!" Theodore A. Baroody, N.D., D.C., Ph.D.

Acidosis
Acidosis is a condition in which the body chemistry becomes imbalanced and overly acidic.

- Respiratory Acidosis is an interruption of the acid control of the body by the lungs. In this case your lungs are unable to remove CO2.
  - Possible causes: asthma, bronchitis, obstructed airway, exhaustion, certain drugs, neurological disorders, inadequate ventilation and etc.
- Metabolic Acidosis is an accumulation of acids or lack of alkaline substances in your blood and other body fluids.
  - Possible causes: aspirin overdose, alcoholism, liver failure, kidney failure, diabetes, starvation, anger, stress, fear, fever, chemical exposure and an overly acidic diet.

What Makes Us Acidic?
In general, an acidic state is caused by: high acid forming diets, depleted alkaline mineral stores, stress and negative emotions, medication/drugs, allergies, poor breathing habits, toxic environment, low water intake, excess alcohol and other items.

Consequences of Being Overly Acidic:
- Oxygen deficiency within cells causes negative changes in cellular metabolism (healthy cells depend on oxygen and glucose for energy production), acidity is a predisposing factor for cancer and other illness and enzymes operate within a narrow pH bandwidth and do not operate within an acidic environment.
- Rheumatoid arthritis, lupus, tuberculosis, osteoporosis, elevated blood pressure, cancer, heart disease, kidney and gall stones, tooth decay, weight problems, immune deficiency, low energy, chronic fatigued, premature aging, and nearly all degenerative disease.

Alkalosis
Alkalosis is a condition in which the fluids of the body are too alkaline. This is less common than acidosis.

Symptoms of Alkalosis: Sore muscles, creaking joints, bursitis, drowsiness, protruding eyes, hypertension, seizures, edema, allergies, night cramps, asthma, chronic indigestion, vomiting, thick blood, dry stools, menstrual problems, thickening of the skin, bone and heel spurs from calcium build up and more.

What makes Us Overly Alkaline?

Most diuretic therapies, excessive intake of alkaline drugs (those for heartburn, ulcer & reflux), excessive vomiting, diarrhea, excessive secretion of aldosterone by the adrenal cortex which can occur when sodium is severely limited and others.

Maintaining Acid and Alkaline Balance
Both alkalosis and acidosis disrupt normal metabolic function and disallow the normal function of critical enzymes. It is critical to regain alkaline balance and achieve a daily ideal range between 7.35 to 7.45. Any readings outside of this range lead to some of the above mentioned scenarios.

Steps To Restoring Acidosis Balance:
Concentrate on the following steps if your saliva or urine shows an acidic or alkalosis state over the course of 7 readings during 1 week.

- Consume the following 3 times a day
  - 8 oz. pure water – pinch sea salt – 1/8 tsp. baking soda – 8 drops trace minerals
- Additional items: Detoxify your body, consume alkaline forming foods, consume coral calcium – magnesium – and potassium supplements, practice meditation – yoga – and deep breathing techniques, get fresh air, practice a 80% to 90% raw diet, drink alkaline water, ingest daily green food supplements, perform oxygen / ozone therapy, ingest daily vegetable juicing, ingest sodium bicarbonate anytime a high acid state may be induced (2 hr after a large meal, 1-2 hr after alcohol) avoid overdosing to avoid alkalosis.

Steps To Restoring Alkalosis:
Though much less common, alkalosis must also be corrected. To regain balance from an overly alkaline state perform the following steps temporarily until balance is restored.

- Check kidney function to ensure they are working properly, supplement with MSM – B-Complex – betaine hydrochloride, temporarily focus on healthy acid-forming foods (about 80%), avoid antacids, lower sodium intake, and check pH daily and continue until pH levels have normalized.

Acid / Alkaline Forming Foods	
Not a Comprehensive List - Find more info @ http://www.thewolfeclinic.com/acidalkfoods.html	
Alkalizing Foods	**Acidic Foods**

Vegetables	Mushrooms	Other	Protein	Grains	Other
Garlic	Lettuce	Stevia	Beef	Rice Cakes	Pasta
Asparagus	Eggplant	Curry	Carp	Amaranth	Distilled
Fermented	Chlorella	Sea Salt	Clams	Barley	Vinegar
Veggies	Rutabaga	All Herbs	Fish	Buckwheat	Wheat
Watercress	Alfalfa	Miso	Lamb	Corn	Germ
Beets	Spirulina	Cinnamon	Salmon	Oats	Beer
Broccoli		Mustard	Tuna	Quinoa	Hard
Brussel	**Fruits**	Maitake		Spelt	Liquor
Sprouts	Apple	Nori	**Fats / Oils**	Kamut	Wine
Cabbage	Apricot	Daikon	Avocado	Wheat	Chemicals
Cauliflower	Figs	Shitake	Oil	Hemp	Drugs,
Eggplant	Dates	Kombu	Hemp Oil	Seed Fiber	Medicinal
Kale	Avocado	Reishi	Flax Oil		Drugs,
Mustard	Banana	Wakame	Safflower	**Beans**	Psychedelic
Greens		Apple	Oil	Black	Herbicides
Dulce	**Protein**	Cider	Canola Oil	Beans	Dairy,
Dandelion	Sprouted	Vinegar		Chick Peas	cheese,
Greens	Seeds	Bee Pollen	**Nut**	Lentils	milk
Sea	Flax Seeds	ProBiotics	**Butters**	Pinto	
Veggies	Egg Whites	Veggie	Cashews	Beans	
Wild	Whey	Juice	Brazil Nuts	Lima	
Greens	Protein	Kombucha	Peanuts	Beans	
Edible	Tofu	Herb Teas	Pecans	White	
Flowers	Tempeh	Green Tea	Tahini	Beans	
Onions		Lecithin		Green Peas	
			Fruits	Red Beans	
			Cranberries	Rice Milk	
				Almond	
				Milk	

PHYSICAL FITNESS STEPS

As previously mentioned although eating properly is the first and best step toward regaining your health and achieving optimal performance, it is not the last or only step.

Achieving a healthy balance both on the inside and outside includes several facets. Knowing, understanding and implementing the philosophy of "moving your body" or "working out" is the second most important aspect of regaining your health. I spoke of two aspects to working out, "resistance training" and "cardio training" earlier, but those are not the only two workout styles. Working outdoors, swimming, bike riding, calisthenics, resistance training, jogging, yoga, Pilates, rowing, isometrics, dancing, playing sports, running, aerobics and many others are all excellent ways to get your body back into great shape.

Earlier I spoke of "resistance and HIIT cardio" training because I believe these are the two most important ways to improve your body structure. But they are not necessarily the most fun.

That being stated, I believe the most important element of moving your body is to have fun while you are doing it.

So, whatever way you decide to move your body be sure to do so 3 to 5 times a week. Each workout session should last at least between 20 to 50 minutes. Your cardio workouts should be high intensity in nature.

Step 11: Stretch - 5 to 7 Days a Week

Stretching is one of the most overlooked aspects of a workout program / active lifestyle. The reality is that our bodies are designed to move on a near constant basis. But modern lifestyles have drastically changed human behavior and routines to a more sedentary lifestyle.

Hard physical labor has been replaced with more sedentary "mental" work styles which involve sitting at desk or standing in one place for extended periods of time.

A way to combat this sedentary lifestyle is to get up and MOVE. Take a walk, do some pushups and yes even stretch. And always, always- it is important to stretch your body before, during and after every workout. Stretching will keep your body warm and lubricated and it will help reduce injuries.

There are several ways to stretch. There is static stretching and ballistic stretching.

Static stretching is the typical method of stretching. Usually it is longer in duration lasting 30 to 60 seconds during each stretch. Ballistic stretching is the style Olympic swimmers use to warm up. They swing their arms back and forth very rapidly but smoothly to avoid injury. Both techniques work. But I recommend sticking mostly to the static technique and then add ballistic occasionally.

Stretching Helps With:
- Reduces muscle tension
- Increases range of motion
- Increases flexibility

Stretching Tips
- Spend 10 – 30 seconds in each stretch. Don't bounce.
- Along with stretching I recommend monthly or bi-monthly massage therapy. Deep massage helps the body eliminate lactic acid build up from weight training or other intense muscle activity.
- I also feel that a good preventative is to schedule chiropractic alignments.

Step 12: "Cardio" – Perform 3 to 5 Days a Week

"Cardio" refers to cardiovascular, also known as aerobic exercise is any physical exercise that improves one's cardiovascular or "oxygen" system resulting in a stronger heart, improved blood flow, improved lung capacity, more oxygen entered into the blood stream. Aerobic means "with oxygen" and refers to the use of oxygen in the body's metabolic or energy-generating process. Many types of exercise like swimming, dancing, running, biking, and plyometrics are aerobic, and by definition are performed at moderate levels of intensity for extended periods of time.

Cardio based exercises are the bane of existence for many, but yet an awesome endorphin high for others! Cardio exercises are both loved and hated worldwide.

But regardless of your love / hate relationship with cardio, there is no doubt that if applied properly, cardio is very good for your body and your mind!

Here's even better news. It was previously thought that cardio workouts needed to be long and tedious. But that is no longer the case. Modern training advice and scientific technology has shown us that there is a very large array of cardio exercises that require only 20 minutes to perform and can reduce fat stores by over 300%

This style of training is called HIIT or High Intensity Interval Training. Think of it this way. Run / swim / bike / dance / roller blade / aerobic workouts and etc. at a brisk rate (after a proper warm up of course) for about 60 seconds then sprint for about 30 to 60 seconds. Back off and repeat this sequence for as long as you can. No more than 20 minutes is normally needed. The above is not a 100% scientific definition, just a basic description.

Many programs I offer like Insanity, Turbo Jam and Turbo Fire are designed as HIIT training styles and will give you intense HIIT fat reductions. HIIT style training is more intense but the results are well worth the efforts!

Cardio Exercise:
- Burns fat
- Elevates heart rate – i.e. builds a stronger heart
- Tones muscles
- Helps clean the Lymphatic system
- Builds stamina

Step 13: Resistance Training – Perform 3 to 5 Days a Week

The most well known resistance training is Weight Training. This includes using dumbbells, barbells, fluids, pressurized air, elastic devices, springs, and a host of other devices designed to provide external resistance to one's musculoskeletal system. There are also several special forms of resistance training which are known as light training. Running, swimming, plyometrics, dance, calisthenics are all special workout forms, all of which are designed to strengthen the body.

With regards to getting in great shape, the idea to hit the gym usually pops into mind. This thought of joining a gym prevents millions of people from achieving a healthy body. Over the years I have heard hundreds of people tell me why they cannot make it to the gym. Have you ever heard any of the following excuses? "I can't afford it", "I don't want to look beefy", "I don't have time", "I have children"?

But there is good news! You don't have to join the gym to get in great shape. The term working out just means MOVE YOUR BODY or GET TO WORK, not, get to the gym! In some parts of the world people still move their bodies from sunrise to sunset. However, in more developed communities manual labor has been replaced by machines, robots and computers.

So what is a person to do? The answer is simple. Start using your body! In the great outdoors preferably! Find something you love like playing tennis, dancing or gardening and do it.

Here are just a few reasons why working out is the second most important element to improving your health.

- Helps to reduce the loss of muscle tissue as you get older. Did you know that on the average we lose 7% of lean muscle mass every 10 years?
- Helps to maintain a stable metabolism. For every one pound of muscle lost, your basal metabolic rate is lowered by fifty calories per day. This means that as you lose muscle you would have to automatically reduce how much you eat. This is impossible to maintain effectively and it is not healthy.
- Helps to maintain bone density
- Helps to maintain flexibility
- Helps to maintain a youthful look
- Helps to maintain a good posture
- Helps to maintain circulation
- Helps to maintain a healthy heart. And in doing so creates greater blood flow to the extremities allowing individuals to reduce their risk of cancer, heart disease and diabetes.

Now what happens if you cannot get outside or make it to your local gym or perhaps you cannot think of a physical activity that suits you? Don't worry about it because I can help! I have an alternative for you.

Visit www.livingonhighspeed.com for details. I have over 130 workout programs all of which can be used in the comfort of your home. 90 of these programs have resistance based training concepts. I probably have something to fit your particular need or desire.

Step 14: Sunshine

Superman, the Man of Steel from Krypton, used the power of the sun to super charge his body and so can you.

Think the sun is bad? Think again! From the dawn of time the sun has been worshipped by almost every society because the sun brings life to Earth. But all experts old and new like the Mayans, Egyptians, Aztecs, farmers and modern scientists realized that the sun is a double-edged sword. The sun can be the bringer of life or the kiss of death depending on the way we use it or how long we enjoy it.

For human and Kryptonian bodies the most important feature of the sun is how our body handles it. Like the son of Krypton, your body uses the sun as a re-charge system. There are many beneficial attributes but the creation of Vitamin D is the most important. Under the action of solar rays, your skin synthesizes vitamin D. Vitamin D facilitates the absorption of calcium and other key nutrients that help keep bones strong and dense.

It is also known that multiple compounds use vitamin D to help your body fight disease. And research shows that sunshine and vitamin D impede the development of some cancer cells. Thus regular and controlled exposure to the sun has a preventive effect against cancer of colon, breast, leukemia, lymphomas and other cancer types.

Moderate exposure to the sun brightens the skin and generates a healthy look and increased elasticity.

Other attributes of correct sun exposure include:

1. Sunlight kills microbes and mold. Place a strawberry in your refrigerator and place one outside in the sun. You will quickly see that the one outside does not develop any mold. Yet the one in the refrigerator will be covered in mold in just a few days. That's why it is important to put out in the sun household items that cannot be washed regularly.
2. Sunlight improves our mood and fights off SAD (Seasonal Affective Disorder). Sunlight helps in cases of chronic or acute depression by stimulating the synthesis of endorphins (feel-good hormones). Lack of sunshine in the winter-time has been attributed to depression in the cold and dark days of the winter.
3. Sunlight aids against insomnia. Daytime exposure to sunlight increases the melatonin production during the night. This hormone helps regulate the sleep.
4. Sunlight strengthens the cardiovascular system. Blood circulation is improved, the pulse, arterial pressure, moderately high glycemia and cholesterol levels can be normalized.
5. Sunlight helps to improve liver functioning, being effective in treating jaundice.
6. Sunlight aids the kidneys as sun waves favor the elimination of waste products through the skin when we sweat.
7. Sunlight helps with weight-loss by increasing the body's metabolic rate through the stimulation of the thyroid gland.
8. Sunlight eases symptoms of premenstrual syndrome.
9. Sunlight ease the swelling of joints during peaks of inflammation in cases of arthritis.

Have you ever had random spots on your body that felt like you were being poked with a pin or perhaps random areas that were very itchy? These symptoms are likely due to a low level of Vitamin D. Checking for low Vitamin D is very easy for your doctor. Have your vitamin D level checked and if it is low, get out in the sun.

The human body requires a modest amount of sunshine. About 10 to 15 minutes a day will do the trick. Some people will experience improvements in overall functioning within a few days or weeks. Other individuals may require a full 6 months to totally recharge their internal batteries. Stick with it. You will definitely feel like Superman in no time at all!
Now there is no substitute like the sun, but we can also derive

Vitamin D from some of the following food sources:
1. Cod liver oil.
2. Deep sea fish like; mackerel, herring, salmon and sardines.
3. Fresh water fish like; trout and catfish.

I hope this helps. Now, break away from your dungeons and go out into the great outdoors and breathe some fresh air and get some sunshine!

Your body, mind and spirit will appreciate it!

Step 15: Sleep

There is no doubt that sleeping properly makes for a better life. With proper sleep we can think better, relax easier, gain muscle or lose fat much more effectively and many additional documented healthy benefits. Volumes have been written on the subject so I will not bore you with all of the scientific mumbo jumbo.

Typically a person needs around 7 to 8 hours of sleep each day. Also it has been found that less sleep and sometimes even too much sleep can often lead to disease. Research suggesting that people eating a raw diet can sleep less over extended periods of time. I am uncertain of this so I will consider the jury is out on this topic until a later date.

Here are a few benefits of proper sleep:
- We grow while sleeping.
- Napping makes us smarter.
- Sleep helps with cell rebuilding / tissue repair.
- Sleep keeps that youthful look by regulating hormones.
- Sleep may be a weight loss aid.
- Sleep improves your memory.
- Sleep makes you more alert.
- Sleep reduces inflammation (the root cause of many diseases).
- Sleeping makes your heart healthy.

Change Your Mind

Changing your mind may be the single most difficult thing to accomplish. Our learned behavior patterns are years even decades old and require more heavy lifting then even the gym requires.

But many giants in the industry have shown over and over that we can renew our minds and renew our behavior patterns.

In fact, some research suggests that in roughly twenty one days of repeated conditioning your mind will form a new habit.

Also, I sometimes find a fine line between what steps should be in the "Change Your Mind" section as compared to the "Change Your Energy" section. In the end they both are closely intertwined.

Step 16: Learn To Quiet Your Mind

Meditation has long been a major central point of spiritual leaders and gurus across the globe. Most religious organizations and many scientists also recognize the value of meditation.

In simple terms meditating is silencing the continual thoughts that are ever present in your mind. Let me illustrate: Have you ever seen someone walking down the street talking to themselves? For the most part the world thinks people who talk out loud to themselves are crazy. But the reality is that all of us "talk" to ourselves. But most of us do so inside of our heads. "*Did I leave the iron on, are the kids okay, the price of gas is crazy, can I pay my bills this month, I hate myself, I hate them, they are strange looking.*" and on and on and on. I dare say most people do this more often then they realize. Practicing meditation on a daily basis is a discipline to cease this internal self talk.

Meditating supports great health by de-stressing your body but it also helps to control impulses and urges of your mind, learned behaviors and your ego as well as deepening your bond with the universe. One of the most important aspects of deep meditation is helping you to hear and understand your inner voice.

Not your ego voice, but your inner voice. Your inner voice will never steer you in the wrong direction, but your ego voice will.

There are many books and trainers available that describe various forms of meditation. Find the book or meditation trainer that meets your meditation style and start implementing as soon as possible. I often refer to this title, <u>Where Ever You Go There You Are</u> by Jon Kabat-Zinn. This book teaches daily meditation habits which can be used calm the mind even on the go or during hectic/busy times.

Here is a simple yet effective mediation practice that I use on a daily basis:
- Get somewhere quiet (no phones, no crying babies, no beeping computers or TVs).
- Sit or lay in a comfortable position (a position that you can comfortably maintain for about fifteen minutes).
- Close your eyes and start deep breathing exercises.
- Focus on one of the following to help keep your mind free and clear of straying thoughts:
  o A blank black screen
  o A flame
- Keep your focus on one of those items and do your best to not think about anything. When a stray thought of any type comes into your mind simply refocus and concentrate on the object in your mind (the flame or the black screen).
- Continue to breathe deep through the entire exercise. I also find it easier to concentrate on my breathing if stray thoughts start to enter my mind.

The practice of meditating may seem difficult in the beginning and you may only be able to focus for a couple of seconds or a few minutes at a time. But if you practice this daily, it will become easier and easier to quiet your mind and meditate as the days and weeks progress.

Step 17: Deep Breathing

Proper deep breathing goes hand in hand with meditation practices. Studies reveal that America is a nation of shallow breathers. This is a causal factor for some of our diseases and for being disconnected from proper meditation and being very stressed. Do not underestimate how important it is to breathe correctly. Breathing correctly is important for living longer, helping your body to fight the good fight to keep you healthy, keeping you at your best and maintaining a balanced mood. Take a look at the following benefits to see why you should make breathing correctly part of your everyday living.

1. Breathing Detoxifies Your Body.

Your body is designed to release toxins through breathing. Unlike our circulatory system, the lymph system does not have a pump to push the lymph fluids. Instead, the lymph system requires the muscular movement which is created by breathing and movement. Also when you exhale air from your body you release carbon dioxide that has been passed through from your bloodstream into your lungs. Carbon dioxide is a natural waste of your body's metabolism.

2. Breathing Relaxes Your Body & Mind.

Breathing relaxes the body and provides oxygen that your body needs. When you are tense, angry, scared or stressed, the body constricts and your muscles get tight and your breathing becomes shallow. Thus tension builds! High or elevating anxiety levels can often be controlled by purposeful deep and slow breathing this will also help to bring mental clarity and deeper insights and understanding. Deep controlled breathing can also help to clear and release emotional anguish and discomfort. If done properly, breathing can help you concentrate on this present moment and not let your mind or emotions get the best of you.

3. Breathing Massages Your Insides.

The movements of the diaphragm during deep breathing exercise massages your stomach, small intestine, liver and pancreas and the heart. Massage is effective at detoxing your muscles, keeps you limber and facilitates the repair and re-growth cycle of your muscles.

4. Breathing Builds Muscle.

Muscles need oxygen. Breathing is the oxygenation process to all of the cells in your body. Yet another reason to breathe properly is to improve circulation and tone your abdominal muscles.

5. Breathing Supports the Immune System.

Oxygen travels through your bloodstream by attaching to hemoglobin in your red blood cells. This helps your body to properly handle / convert / absorb nutrients and vitamins.

6. Breathing Improves Posture.

Good breathing techniques over a sustained period of time will encourage good posture. Correct posture and breathing support multiple organ functions.

7. Breathing Improves The Digestive Process.

   The digestive organs such as the stomach receive more life giving oxygen.

8. Breathing Helps the Nervous System.

   The brain, spinal cord and nerves are more nourished when you breath deeply.

9. Breathing Strengthens the Lungs & Heart.

   The heart & lungs are muscle. Muscles love to be worked out and the lungs are no exception. Strong deep breathing makes the lungs healthy and powerful. And if you mix proper breathing with good cardio then you are sure to avoid future respiratory problems. Stronger lungs are more efficient, which means more oxygen is brought into contact with blood sent to the lungs by the heart. So, the heart doesn't have to work as hard to deliver oxygen to the tissues. Lastly, deep breathing leads to a greater pressure differential in the lungs, which leads to an increase in the circulation. Thus the heart can rest a little.

10. Breathing Keeps The Weight Off.

    If you are overweight, the extra oxygen burns up the excess fat more efficiently. If   you are underweight, the extra oxygen feeds the starving tissues and glands.

11. Breathing Boosts Energy Levels.

    Improves stamina and deep breathing increase pleasure-inducing neuro-chemicals in   the brain to elevate moods and combat physical pain.

12. Breathing Aids Meditation.

Breathing Exercises

In order to breathe properly you need to breathe deeply into your abdomen not just your chest. Breathing exercises should be deep, slow, rhythmic and in through the nose not through the mouth. But it is acceptable to breathe out through your mouth.

1. Inhale through your nose, expanding your belly, while then filling your chest with air for a count of 5 seconds.
2. Hold your breath and count to five.
3. Exhale fully from through a slightly parted mouth and feel all your cells releasing waste and emptying all old energy. Exhale to a count of five or ten if your lungs can handle it.

Repeat at least five times during each session.

Set time aside for at least two to three 10 minute segments every day. You can begin with two five minutes segments if you prefer. Practice deep breathing techniques 2 or 3 times a day while at work, in your car, at home or anywhere you can relax or be alone.

Deep Breathing - Practice It Daily

Step 18: Identify Your Trigger Points

A few years ago I saw my first "Dog Whisperer" television episode hosted by Cesar Millan and have been a Dog Whisperer junkie ever since. Presently I do not own a dog.

Cesar has the most direct approach to solving some personal issues that I have ever seen or studied. Yes his training is aimed at dogs, but his principals also apply to you and me.

Here is the basic principal. We all have decision points or trigger points in our lives that occur all day long. When those points occur we have a decision to go left or right, forward or backward, to react positively or react negatively, to be nice or to be mean, to speak softly or speak loudly, to snap or to be silent and so on. How one reacts largely depends on their background, their perception of their background and their ability to remain calm and focused.

Unfortunately, many people react with less than a positive action. Meaning, they "snap" at their family members or perhaps hold a grudge, and become resentful and later "blow up" and hurt or harm someone else around them.

So here is my take on this. We all have ability at that very moment to react differently, to go right instead of left to be quite instead of exploding, to be positive instead of being negative, to not pick up that cigarette or that alcoholic drink. The ability to sense this moment can be very difficult in the beginning but over time you can hone your senses and your skills to react in a different way.

Cesar Millan specializes in observing the canine behavior and identifying the exact moment of a mental shift from calm to alert or aggressive behavior. Cesar is able to redirect the dog's focus from the first thought to another thought within a fraction of a second. This technique is one of the most powerful techniques I have seen to shift one's focus and therefore modify behavior.

This concept of identifying and changing focus points has also benefited many humans. Now the problem is that we do not have a personal "Cesar" or an electronic zapper on our bodies or our minds that will "zap" us when we react negatively. So, it is up to each of us to recognize this within ourselves. By the way, smokers sometimes use an interesting concept of placing a rubber band around their wrist. This technique worked for many smokers to "kick" the habit. One just needs to find that "proper" redirection point that will move you back into a proper thought pattern.

Now this concept of "redirection" applies to all thoughts that you do not think are proper for you and your lifestyle. Not just moments of anger, but other times like allowing sadness to overcome you or moments of infidelity, thoughts of punching your boss and others also apply. In these moments you have a choice to go left or go right. The question is, "are you aware or not?" Do you know how your reactions are affecting your health and others around you?

Read one of Cesar Millan's books. You will not regret it.

Step 19: Learn To Release

Have you ever grabbed something HOT? I know I have. I quickly dropped it. Dropping something hot is our body's a natural protection mechanism. This keeps us from causing major harm to our bodies.

Similarly, your psyche has a built-in mechanism that protects you from any emotional or mental damage. This faint mechanism is difficult to cultivate and must be nurtured. Over time the ability to recognize and follow the path of enlightenment and joy will become much easier.

Unfortunately, most people tend to hold onto emotional damage for far too long. Typically the longer we hold on to emotional harm the "harder" we become. Holding on to negative thoughts and reactions create many negative impacts on the body, mind and the spirit.

Stress is created when we hold too tightly to the harm which was inflicted upon us. Stress causes the body to release cortisol and other chemicals that cause harm if not expunged. It has even been found that DNA can be altered if too much hatred is stored up inside of the body for extended periods. So the next time something happens to you, just drop it. It seriously is that easy. No matter what the harm, no matter what is said, no matter what is done, your health, your sanity and your family's security is worth much more than the damage you will cause to your health.

Hale Dwoskin is founder of the Sedona Method. Hale's course is great at teaching one how to release all current, future and past harmful emotional baggage.

See my website www.livingonhighspeed.com for more details concerning releasing and the Sedona Method.

Step 20: Live In The Now

Living in the "Now" is not much different than meditating, deep breathing or following the releasing techniques or even the trigger point techniques. In fact *"Living in the now, or Living in this present moment* is all of those items wrapped into one teaching concept.

But it is different enough for me to talk about because to truly believe and understand the previously mentioned techniques, one should have a firm grasp on understanding that there is no yesterday and there is no tomorrow. There is only the Now. And in the Now is where you can grasp the understanding of the world around us and even the power of the universe.

You see, *Living in the Now* and not over-reacting but listening to your inner voice and listening to what the natural world is saying will set you free. This may sound easy, but try just for a day to not think about what happen to you in the past or what may happen in the future and bet it will be a stretch to accomplish.

The best teacher in the industry about "Living In The Now or Living In This Present Moment" is Eckhart Tolle.

Step 21: Recreation

Go outside, have some fun and do something you enjoy!
Life is too short to hate your daily activities and exercise programs! Learn to enjoy life to its fullest!

- Relax - cortisol levels will lower.
- Take time to enjoy life and smell the roses (or a flower of your choice).
- Live in *"This Present Moment"* always and your world will change.

Step 22: Grow Something

Growing one's living food has become a lost art form for certain segments of society. Society now relies heavily on grocery stores and shipping companies to provide their daily food. And due to corporate farming practices and big business greed most small, medium and even large farms have been run out of business thus making it even more difficult to find fresh live food from local sources.

Being removed from personal gardens and local farms has resulted in the world's population to become disconnected from planet Earth. This disconnection has caused many problems and perhaps more than I could discuss in this book.

Being disconnected from the Earth means we lose the energy connection the Earth provides this also means we are mostly disconnected from the universe. Many people have lost touch with everything around them and live mostly in their minds. Our days are filled with business thoughts, watching TV, thoughts of what I will be doing tomorrow and so much more.

This is not good!

One way to begin to re-connect is to start growing one's own food. I will discuss this subject further in a later book but for now focus on something easy. Growing something like wheat grass or barley grass or an herb garden can be an easy start. These can be grown in any home or apartment. You could also invest in a Grow Box or an Earth Box. These boxes can be placed in any living environment such as a balcony of a small apartment or any home or office space. If you have land of any size then you have a great opportunity. Use that land and touch the earth and grow something wild!

Your heart and you life force will love you for it!

Step 23: Stress Avoidance

Stress really is avoidable in today's hectic lifestyle. Stress avoidance drastically increases your body's ability to fight off disease and promotes happier healthier lives. But stress seems greatly infused into the American lifestyle.

- Stress depletes water soluble vitamins.
- Stress causes premature aging.
- Stress causes cellular breakdown (disease) and taps into energy stores.
- Stress causes a build-up of cortisol, which is a catabolic agent (meaning it is a carcinogen and it eats away at living tissue).
- Stress causes training plateaus.

So besides moving to a Buddhist Monastery and becoming Buda what are we to do?

Here are a few suggestions to reduce stress:
- Don't over - react to situations.
- Don't over - extend your schedule.
- Don't eat while watching TV.
- Don't discuss stressful issues while eating.

Going further:
- Create an action plan to ID your hot buttons and RELEASE them.
- Rid yourself of as many stressors as possible.
- Start meditating daily.
- Start deep breathing exercises.
- Start an exercise program. (Working out releases health and growth hormones that will help combat stress related cortisol.)
- Create a meal plan that includes more fresh fruits and vegetables.
- Start reading self help books. Reading a chapter or small section each day will reap benefits.

(Recommended reading, The Power Of Now, Where Ever You Go There You Are, The Sedona Method, anything by Wayne Dyer and read a couple of Cesar Millan's books).

You can't avoid stress! But, you can learn to rid its effects from your body, mind and your spirit. But only if you take the time to do so.

Change Your Life Energy

Changing your life energy is more of an ongoing process and a state of mind than anything else.

The most important aspect of changing your energy is to connect with the world around you and to become one with the universe. The benefits of becoming one with the universe are too many to discuss in this one book. But the primary benefit of becoming one with the universe is to know one's self. When you know yourself, you can become a shining beacon of hope for those around you and for yourself. You will be able to follow your passion and nothing will be able to deter you from your path.

The next item is to enhance the ability to listen to your inner voice. This voice comes from the universe, from some ultimate energy or source, or from God. This voice will never steer you wrong.

The last, and to some the most exciting, piece of changing one's internal energy is the amazing ability to attract the life giving positive energy that fills this world and comes from the greater universe. When you are aligned with your purpose and aligned with the proper energy frequency then doors open for you that seem magical. Things and people come your way from seemingly nowhere to support you and provide prosperity to you in many unforeseen ways.

If you would like to learn more about life energy, universal connectedness and higher energy living then refer to publications that discuss some of the following: quantum mechanics, quantum entanglement, the laws of attraction and books written by Louise Hay or Wayne Dwyer and Eckhart Tolle.

As a last comment on this subject, I would also like to let you know that many of the steps in the "Change Your Mind" section are closely related to changing your life energy. These steps are a process of a full life change and work together to help create a better you and a better world.

Step 24: Attitude

Webster's defines attitude as: a feeling or emotion (mental position) toward a fact or state.
- Attitude is a choice, positive or negative.
- What you think about, you bring about.
- It is said that what we fear may come upon us.
- A proverb states: As a man thinketh in his heart, so is he.
- Attitude affects every part of your life: physical, mental and spiritual.
- The words you speak can bring life or death.
- Your attitude is everything.

Here are 4 words you should not allow in your home.
- **Hate** – Just using that word gives you a negative feeling and causes your body to feel tense.
- **Stupid** – This word is not uplifting or edifying
- **Can't** – Why tell yourself you can't do something? Your mind does not know the difference between what is real and what is not real.
- **Problem** – There is no such thing. Why make it into a problem? There are just challenges.

Step 25: Truthfulness

It is said that "Honesty is the best policy". You may ask, "What does being truthful have anything to do with my health?" Lying or untruthfulness affects the body, again, by putting the body in a negative state. When you are not truthful your body has a tendency to tense up. When the body is tense, hormones, chemicals and toxins are released which cause damage to the body over time.

Step 26: Punctuality

Today we live in the busiest and fastest paced society that ever existed. Everyone has a schedule to keep, rushing here and there, racing the clock and snapping at everyone or anything that gets in their way. This is not a very relaxed life.

Being punctual is an important character trait but not at the risk of your health. If you have a problem getting to places on time, LEAVE EARLIER!

Step 27: Forgiveness - Generosity - Love

Forgiveness
Un-forgiveness breeds bitterness and bitterness can breed disease. Having a bitter heart towards someone actually puts your body in a negative state. If you stay in that state for long periods of time or on a regular basis your digestion will be drastically affected causing poor digestion which leads to an entire host of problems.

Generosity
Have you ever given something away and felt good regardless of their reaction. So many people are living their lives as takers. If they only knew what the secret of giving could do in their lives. Free yourself from being tense and un-giving.

Love
Spend your day walking in love and avoiding conflict with others and you will be amazed how much energy you will have left at the end of the day. You will have less stressed out days. You will be healthier and more fun to be around.

Step 28: Practice Energy Exercises

The more than 60 trillion cells that reside within your body all are powered with an energy source. This energy source is thought by nearly all scientist, quantum mechanics, spiritual and religious gurus to be connected at a quantum level to the Earth and even to the universe around us.

This connection has been proven in scientific laboratories and to some extent proven in prayer circles, churches, synagogues, mosques and energy consciousness classes like QiGong.

All of humanity refers to this energy by a different name: God, Allah, The Holy Spirit, Mother Earth, Quantum Energy, Universal Energy and thousands of other names.

Regardless of your belief and the name you call it, there is no doubt that we should cleanse our life energy and add new clean energy as often as possible just as we do with our bodies and our cars.

By practicing all of the steps in both the Mind and Energy sections, one can cleanse & renew their energies. Here are additional practices to conclude this section of the LOHS Change Your Life steps.

1. **Prayer** – One of the first and most prevalent energy changers on the planet is prayer. Every religion and every spiritual guru guides us through prayer. Many also teach us to direct our prayers. Prayer has been proven to be effective especially with corporate or mass prayer. Even scientist can track "electrical" changes in atmosphere during mass, unified prayers.
    a. It is important to note that prayer has been shown to be more effective when coupled with meditation and fasting.
2. **Energy Movements** – There are several energy-based exercise programs available across the globe. Most of these programs are based on old Eastern concepts. Most of these concepts have a belief that there is energy residing within us.
    a. **QiGong** – Is translated from the Chinese to mean "energy cultivation" or "working with the life energy." Qigong is an ancient Chinese system of postures, exercises, breathing techniques, and meditations. Its techniques are designed to improve and enhance the body's *qi*. According to traditional Chinese philosophy, qi is the fundamental life energy responsible for health and vitality.

    Qigong may be used as a daily routine to increase overall health and well-   being, as well as for disease prevention and longevity. It can be used to increase energy and reduce stress. In China, Qigong is used in conjunction with other medical therapies for many chronic conditions including asthma,   allergies, AIDS, cancer, headaches, hypertension, depression, mental illness,   strokes, heart disease, and obesity.
    b. **Reiki** – The word Reiki is made of two Japanese words - Rei which means "God's Wisdom or the Higher Power" and Ki which

is "life force energy". So Reiki is actually "spiritually guided life force energy".

An amazingly simple technique to learn, the ability to use Reiki is not taught in the usual sense, but is transferred to the student during a Reiki class.

Are you ready to put these steps into an action plan?

Join the Vortex Zone at www.livingonhighspeed.com and choose one of the following exciting challenge programs:
- Living On High Speed Life Challenge

You can take charge of changing your life and forever be changed!

Part 8

Creating A High Speed World

Chapter 13

Living On High Speed Together

Living On High Speed is more than a book, it is more than a web site, and it is more than a cute name. Living On High Speed is a total wellness community that offers teaching on all facets of health and wellness.

Let Living On High Speed teach you how to combine all facets of wellness into a comprehensive life changing plan.

Change Your Body / Change Your Mind / Change Your Energy and Change Your Life.

Are you ready to change your life? If yes is the answer, then let's get busy!

- **Vortex Zone** – The **Vortex Zone** is an exciting new endeavor I have created to help you become your best. As a **Vortex Zone** member you will have access to some of the following benefits:
  - Daily motivational and educational email reminders
  - Exclusive weekly fun and entertaining educational videos that expand on each point of *Living On High Speed* book
  - Exclusive Wellness Blog sessions with myself and other like minded health professionals
  - Exclusive Video Blog sessions with myself and other like minded health professionals
  - Exclusive rights to join for free the following exciting program
    - Living On High Speed 1 Year Change Your Life Challenge
  - Advanced notice of all future book releases
  - 25% discount on all future books and service orders I offer

Find the **Vortex Zone** at www.livingonhighspeed.com

- **Follow us @ www.LivingOnHighSpeed.com**

Change Your Body / Change Your Mind / Change Your Energy / Change Your Life

Do you want more? Would you like to help America regain its health? I hope so, because the American health and wellness industry and the wellness movement has been "losing" the battle. The battle I am talking about is the battle for health of the American population in general. Each year the nation is becoming more obese and more people are dying from disease that can be controlled by wellness techniques.

There are many reasons we are losing this battle. A lack of personal self control, chemical addictions, hectic lifestyles, poor time management skills and more are all contributing factors. But the primary reason we are losing the battle is "lack of unification". The two areas of lack of unification are:
1. Wellness Educators
2. American Consumers (that's all of us by the way)

There are three areas that fuel this "lack of unification".
1. Confusion
    a. Americans are confused by all of the choices, confused by all of the misguided marketing and confused by misguided and sometimes false medical claims from wellness companies, the medical community and government agencies.
2. Greed & Survival
    a. Small and medium sized businesses are in a daily fight for their survival. Inflation and the drastic increase in goods and services have made it difficult for entrepreneurs to make an honest profit. Beating the competition at any expense is all too often commonplace in the health & wellness field. Most wellness professionals promote only their products / books/ services often telling consumers that this diet, this supplement or this program is the BEST. This has caused severe confusion and sometimes it even causes tension and disbelief.
3. Control & Corruption
    a. This disjointed "survival mode" has allowed the medical, insurance, chemical, and pharmaceutical industries to become the largest and most powerful entities in the world. While the wellness

industry and wellness professionals were scampering for new customers and bickering between each other about what diet is best, what supplement is best and even what books were best, the medical, pharmaceutical, chemical and insurance agencies were lobbying Congress, infiltrating Congress, the FDA, OSHA, USDA, the Supreme Court and many additional government agencies. These entities now control most governmental organizations and have influenced massive legislation to be written in their favor.

This has caused an imbalance in America and in the world at large. Major corporations are growing richer and richer as each year passes.

This will not always be the case. I am confident that if enough people band together to defend themselves against governmental and corporate control then all of our freedoms and liberties can become secured.

Here are a few ways we can unify and turn things around.
- Use Your Purchasing Power Wisely.
- Educate Yourself.
- Direct Your Life.
  - Change Your Energy and Teach Others To Do the Same.
- Get "Tiny". – Decrease materialism and decrease your debt load.
- Join Like Minded Organizations and Become Active.

Purchasing Power – Money is "king". So, use your wallets to speak for you. These businesses became large and powerful due to almost unlimited funding. Their money came from you! Use your purchasing power to redirect sales away from these corporate giants and start purchasing food and other necessities direct from local farmers and small business owners.

Educate Yourself – Turn your televisions sets from corporate sponsored / censored media and start reading and listening to the independent press and freedom fighters whose intentions are to free us from the rule and reign of the ruling elite class.

Here are a few of my favorite freedom fighters:
- Health Freedom Fighters – David Wolfe, Markus Rothkranz, Gary Null and many others.
- Conspiracy Freedom Fighters – Kevin Trudeau, Alex Jones, Jesse Ventura and many others.

Direct Your Life – It's an amazing feeling to be confident and secure about your health and your future. Yet this security and confidence alludes many. The good news is that there are many ways to secure your life. The most important is not to "buy the "hype". Meaning stop listening to corporate commercial propaganda. In the best case scenario, corporate entities broadcast *slanted* messages to increase your purchases of their products. In the worst case scenario, corporate entities control your life with false messages.

In addition to the corporate and media hype, one must also learn to stop relying on the medical institution as your health care provider. The medical industry is actually the sickness industry. More importantly, they are also a for profit industry. Thus, their primary directive is to earn a profit at your expense. They are trained in emergency management and identifying when you are sick but they are not trained in what it takes to improve your health. So do your research and find local alternative health care providers. This includes, but is certainly not limited to, some of the following:

- Fitness trainers, nutrition counselors, massage therapists, yoga instructors, QiGong instructors, raw food nutritionist, detox specialist, acupuncturists, accupressurists, chiropractors, Naturopaths', meditation experts and many other natural wellness providers.

Also you can take charge of your life and help change the world by doing one of the following:

- Become A Certified Wellness Expert – Have you ever wanted to become a Certified Nutritionist, Raw Food Nutritionist, Sports Nutritionist, certified Life Coach? If these fields interest you, then go to my website www.livingonhighspeed.com to learn how you can join the ranks as a wellness educator!
- Become A Fitness Coach – Would you like to help people get in shape? Is your time and money limited? Instead of becoming a certified fitness instructor, consider becoming a Team Beach Body coach. You would have the re-sell rights to America's top workout programs like P90X, Insanity, Hip Hop Abs, Turbo Jam, Turbo Fire and more. Check out my website www.livingonhighspeed.com to learn more about this exciting opportunity.

Get Tiny – No, I do not mean lose weight. Instead I mean stop your desire to own all the toys and gadgets the world has to offer. This unquenchable materialism has driven people to an unhealthy level of consumerism. We buy way too much, way too often. We often live on credit and live in houses that are much bigger than we need. We buy and eat too much food and own too many creature comforts and live extravagant lifestyles.

If you pay off your credit cards, if you pay off your homes, if you stop buying every latest new toy that comes on the market, if you grow your own food and become self sustaining, then you have made the largest statement to the world that you are using your life and purchasing power for the betterment of mankind and not for the betterment of the corporate consumer machine. You have freed yourself from the "machine" and become tiny.

Join Like Minded Organizations & Become Active – Remember the old saying that "Together we stand but divided we fall"? Well, there is no doubt that finding like minded people and banning together is one of the most influential ways to make a change. There are many organizations that are fighting the good fight but they all need your help. So find a like minded organization that you can support with your time or your funding and start changing the world!

Edmond Burke once stated: "All that is necessary for the triumph of evil is that good men do nothing".

Let's not let evil triumph. Together we can create a shift in human evolution. We just need to step out of our boxes, become good men and women who do something. When you do, the world will respond.

Change Your Body / Change Your Mind / Change Your Energy / Change Your Life

Change The World

Part 9

Warning – Sudden Death May Occur

This last section is dedicated to my mother and to well over 250,000 that are killed by the medical profession each year. While *Living On High Speed* is not directly about this subject, I want for you to know that I will be creating yet another educational book sometime in the near future on this subject.

The following is a small section from this future book:

The word "iatrogenic" comes from the Greek roots "iatros" meaning "the healer or physician" + "gennan" meaning "as a product of" = due to the doctor.

Some *iatrogenic errors* are easily identified, such as a complication following a surgical procedure. Some errors are less obvious and require significant investigation to identify, such as complex drug interactions.

Direct causes of iatrogenesis include: medical errors, negligence, social control and the adverse effects or interactions of prescription drugs. In the United States an estimated 98,000 to 325,000 deaths per year may be attributed to iatrogenesis making the medical establishment (hospitals, emergency rooms, pharmaceutical companies, doctors, nurses and more) to be the ***third leading cause of death*** in the United States. These numbers are directly related to death and do not include the numbers related to the many other negative effects of Iatrogenesis such as disability, injuries and discomfort that are also associated to Iatrogenesis.

The total death count is hard to pin down for many reasons, but the primary reason these facts are hidden and not being broadcast by the media or government are "corruption".

Think about it. If a car manufacture created a car that killed 98,000 people every year then you could be sure that the car would be recalled and the company would be tied up in law suits. Likewise, if a nutritional supplement killed the same number of people then the supplement company would be shut down and possibly the CEO and the lead scientists would be sued, fired or arrested.

Yet the medical profession, doctors and pharmaceutical companies are allowed to kill Americans every single year. Not only are they allowed to kill but I would say they are encouraged to do so. Doctors, medical and big pharmaceutical board members, CEOs, lobbyist and more are paid high income and bonus money each year to do the same. In-fact, the medical institution is the highest paid industry in the nation and they use this money to control the laws and legislations that will protect them and their interest.

Another fact that is all too often overlooked is the "war" statistics. For instance, the total ten year casualty count for both the Iraq war and the Afghanistan war is slightly over 6,990. The total casualty count for the 10 year Vietnam "war" conflict is a little over 58,236.

Put into perspective, the medical profession and all supporters that protect these organizations such as congressmen, lobbyist and the media are responsible for more American deaths than both terrorist and war put together.

This might be tolerable if it resulted in better health, but does it? Out of 13 countries in a recent comparison, the United States ranks an average of 12th (second from the bottom) for 16 available health indicators. More specifically, the ranking of the U.S. on several indicators was:
- 13th (last) for low-birth-weight percentages
- 13th for neonatal mortality and infant mortality overall[14]
- 11th for post-neonatal mortality
- 13th for years of potential life lost (excluding external causes)
- 11th for life expectancy, at 1 year for females, 12th for males
- 10th for life expectancy, at 15 years for females, 12th for males
- 10th for life expectancy, at 40 years for females, 9th for males
- 7th for life expectancy, at 65 years for females, 7th for males
- 3rd for life expectancy, at 80 years for females, 3rd for males
- 10th for age-adjusted mortality
- The poor performance of the U.S. was recently confirmed by a World Health Organization study which used different data and ranked the United States as 15th among 25 industrialized countries.

The point?

AVOID THE MEDICAL ESTABLISHMENT!

Don't get me wrong. There are instances when the medical institution is needed and beneficial. Medical professionals are needed for emergencies and in rare cases when your body is unable to heal itself from a disease.

Other than that, your body can and will heal itself of most disease as long as you give it the nutrients, proper breathing, meditation (to reverse stress and connect with the electrical universal connection), rest, workouts (to release stress and many growth and repair hormones), sunlight and many other exciting and helpful items.

I have a question for you. Would you eat food if it came with any of the following side effect: "rash; hives; itching; difficulty breathing; tightness in the chest; swelling of the mouth, face, lips, or tongue; joint pain; purple or brownish red spots on the skin); behavior changes (eg, aggression, hostility); blurred vision or other vision problems; chest pain; confusion; dark urine; fainting; fast or irregular heartbeat; fever, chills, or sore throat; hallucinations; mental or mood changes (eg, agitation, anxiety, depression, irritability, persistent crying, unusual sadness); one-sided weakness; seizures; severe or persistent dizziness or headache; shortness of breath; slurred speech; suicidal thoughts or attempts; uncontrolled speech or muscle movements; yellowing of the eyes or skin"?

Probably not. In-fact if there were such a food that caused even a few of these symptoms, I can guarantee you it would be pulled off of store shelves. Yet this list is associated with a pharmaceutical medication that hundreds of thousands of American parents give their children every single day. You see, the above side effects are the side effects that I copied from the Ritalin paperwork.

Sadly the tragedy of iatrogenisis does not stop at just a casualty count. Iatrogenic errors also account for yet another 1.7 million adverse injuries and other minor or major side effects.

How do we avoid this?

STAY AWAY FROM HOSPITALS, PHARMACUETICAL DRUGS and even some MEDICAL PROFESSIONALS.

You accomplish this by keeping your body fit and healthy by eating well, working out and avoid the toxic things in life!

This is not a sure fired answer and there are no 100% guarantees to keep you out of harm's way. It is however well known that you can keep yourself healthy and fit if you set your mind to it. And if you do, then perhaps just maybe you can avoid the clause "sudden death may occur" Let's stop the madness, get off the drugs and change our lives!

Don't let big business and media control you! Take control of your life and make a change for the better and who knows, perhaps you will live a longer healthy and happier life for it!

About The Author

Scott Black is a health educator who believes in an individual's right to control their lifelong health and "Total Wellness". He is passionate about people holding corporations and government agencies accountable to make available in the national marketplace an affordable diversity of healthy choices.

Since there is no "magic pill" and no "one size fits all" program, Scott teaches that achieving total wellness is a balancing act that combines all aspects of *Body, Mind and Energy* training.

His quest to become a life changer "sprouted" due to witnessing his youthful mother (38 years old) lose her health & life to cancer. Scott continues to educate himself, his family and friends and many others on how to live and enjoy total wellness in this fast paced modern life.

While Scott served as a weapons engineer instructor in Italy for the U.S. Air Force, he became a personal trainer & sports nutritionist and helped U.S. military members and Italian civilians.

Later, while being an executive trainer in several American corporations, Scott earned certifications as a Raw Nutritionist, Certified Nutrition Consultant and Detox Specialist.

After 10 years Scott left "Corporate America" to become a full time wellness business owner providing one-on-one personal wellness training, wellness seminars, live food cooking demonstrations, Vita-Mix demonstrations, call -to-action events, on-line wellness support, wellness videos, books, blogs, newsletters and more.

Known as Coach Scott to friends and clients, Scott is an author, blogger and a wellness video producer. He has been a guest speaker on many on-line radio shows and provides community support through his website: www.livingonhighspeed.com

Scott resides in South Florida with his wife and business partner Barbara.

Made in the USA
Charleston, SC
07 March 2014